PROBLEMS AND METHODS IN THE HISTORY OF MEDICINE

THE WELLCOME INSTITUTE SERIES IN THE
HISTORY OF MEDICINE

Edited by W.F. Bynum and Roy Porter, The Wellcome
Institute

Medical Fringe and Medical Orthodoxy, 1750–1850
W.F. Bynum and Roy Porter

Florence Nightingale and the Nursing Legacy
Monica Baly

Social Hygiene in Twentieth Century Britain
Greta Jones

In Preparation

Living and Dying in London
Edited by W.F. Bynum

PROBLEMS
AND METHODS
IN THE HISTORY
OF MEDICINE

Edited by Roy Porter and Andrew Wear

CROOM HELM
London ● New York ● Sydney

© 1987 Roy Porter and Andrew Wear
Croom Helm Ltd, Provident House, Burrell Row,
Beckenham, Kent BR3 1AT

Croom Helm Australia Pty Ltd, Suite 4, 6th Floor,
64–76 Kippax Street, Surry Hills, NSW 2010, Australia

Published in the USA by
Croom Helm in association with Methuen, Inc.
29 West 35th Street
New York, NY10001

British Library Cataloguing in Publication Data

Problems and methods in this history of medicine.
   — (The Wellcome Institute series in the history of medicine)
   1. Medicine — Historiography
   I. Porter, Roy, 1946–   II. Wear, A.
   III. Series
   610'.72   R131
   ISBN 0–7099–3687–7

Library of Congress Cataloging-in-Publication Data

Problems and methods in the history of medicine.

   (The Wellcome Institute series in the history of
medicine
   1. Medicine — Historiography. I. Porter, Roy,
1946- . II. Wear, A. (Andrew), 1946- .
III. Series. [DNLM: 1. Historiography. 2. History
of Medicine. WZ 345 P962]
R133.P74 1987   610'.9   87-478
ISBN 0-7099-3687-7

Filmset by Mayhew Typesetting, Bristol, England
Printed and bound in Great Britain by
Biddles Ltd, Guildford and King's Lynn

Contents

Notes on Contributors   vi
Acknowledgements   ix
Introduction   1

I   The French Connection   13

  1. Toby Gelfand   The *Annales* and Medical
                                Historiography: *Bilan et
                                Perspectives*   15
  2. J.-P. Goubert   Twenty Years On: Problems
                                of Historical Methodology in
                                the History of Health   40
  3. Colin Jones   Montpellier Medical Students
                                and the Medicalisation of
                                18th-Century France   57
  4. Françoise Loux   Popular Culture and
                                Knowledge of the Body:
                                Infancy and the Medical
                                Anthropologist   81

II   Medical History and Historical Demography   99

  5. Arthur E. Imhof   Methodological Problems in
                                Modern Urban History
                                Writing: Graphic
                                Representations of Urban
                                Mortality 1750–1850   101
  6. E.A. Wrigley   No Death Without Birth:
                                The Implications of English
                                Mortality in the Early
                                Modern Period   133

III Computers and the History of Institutions   151

  7. Anne Digby   Quantitative and Qualitative
                                Perspectives on the Asylum   153
  8. Guenter B. Risse   Hospital History: New
                                Sources and Methods   175

IV   The Qualitative and the Quantitative   205

  9. Michael MacDonald Madness, Suicide, and the
                                Computer   207
  10. Andrew Wear   Interfaces: Perceptions of
                                Health and Illness in Early
                                Modern England   230

Index   257

Notes on Contributors

Anne Digby is at present a Research Fellow at the Institute for Research in the Social Sciences at the University of York, but is moving shortly to be a Research Associate at the Institute of Economics and Statistics in the University of Oxford. She has written extensively on modern British social policy and on the history of medicine. Among her publications are *Pauper Palaces* (Routledge, 1978), *Madness, Morality and Medicine: A Study of the York Retreat, 1796–1914* (Cambridge, 1985), and (with Peter Searby), *Children, School and Society in Nineteenth-Century England* (Macmillan, 1981). Currently, she is working on doctor-patient relationships in the eighteenth and nineteenth centuries.

Toby Gelfand is Professor in the Faculty of Health Sciences, University of Ottawa (Hannah Chair) and the Department of History. Born in Philadelphia in 1942, he took his PhD in the History of Medicine at the Johns Hopkins University. He is the author of *Professionalizing Modern Medicine: Paris Surgeons and Medical Science and Institutions in the 18th Century* (Westport, Conn., Greenwood Press, 1980) and articles in the *Bulletin of the History of Medicine, Medical History, Revue d'Histoire Moderne et Contemporaine, Histoire Sociale-Social History*. His current project is: "The Language of Pathology: Medical Discourse and the Jews in France (1850–1900)".

Jean-Pierre Goubert is Maître de Conférences à l'École des Hautes Etudes en Sciences Sociales (Centre de Recherches Historiques) and Docteur des Lettres (1984), Université de Paris-VII, mention Très Honorable. His principal publications are *Malades et Médecines en Bretagne 1770–1790* (Paris, Klincksieck, 1974); (editor) *Le Médicalisation de la Société Française, 1770–1830* (University of Waterloo, Canada, 1982); *Le Corps Médical et le Changement: 1789 . . .* (in collaboration with Dominique Lorillot) (Toulouse, Privat, 1984), *La Conquête de l'Eau. L'Avènement de la Santé à l'Âge Industriel* (introduction by Emmanuel Le Roy Ladurie) (Paris, Rober Leffont, 1986).

Arthur E. Imhof was born in Switzerland in 1939. He studied history in Zurich, Brussels, Paris and Rome, and obtained his

PhD at the University of Zurich in 1965. He was a Research Fellow of the Swiss National Science Foundation in Scandinavia until 1973, Assistant Professor at the University of Giessen, West Germany, from 1973 to 1975, and he has been Full Professor of Social History at the Friedrich-Meinecke Institute at the Freie Universität, Berlin, since 1975. He has held Guest-Professorships at the École des Hautes Études en Sciences Sociales in Paris, at the Hebrew University of Jerusalem, and at different Universities in Brazil and New Zealand. He was also Visiting Research Fellow of the Japan Society for the Promotion of Science in Tokyo, and at the Institute of Advanced Studies, Research School of Social Sciences, in Canberra, Australia. His publications include *Die Gewonnenen Jahre* (C.H. Beck, 1981); *Die Verlorenen Welten* (C.H. Beck, 1984); and as editor *Der Mensch und sein Körper* (C.H. Beck, 1983).

Colin Jones is Lecturer in History at Exeter University. His research is on French social history from the seventeenth to the early nineteenth century. He is the author of *Charity and 'bienfaisance': the treatment of the poor in the Montpellier region, 1740–1815* (Cambridge, 1982).

Françoise Loux is an anthropologist and head of research at the Centre National de la Recherche Scientifique, France. She works at the Centre d'Ethnologie Française, part of the Musée des Arts et Traditions Populaires, Paris, on the body and its meaning in traditional, rural French Society. Her current research bears on popularisation of theoretical knowledge and charitable medicine in chapbooks; French popular remedies; the transmission of knowledge of the body and nature among mountain guides. Along with health service practitioners she is also engaged in research projects and teaching in the field of 'anthropology and nursing practices'. Her publications include *Sagesse due Corps* (with P. Richard) (G.P. Maisonneuve et Lerose, 1978), *Le Jeune Enfant et Son Corps dans la Médecine Traditionelle* (Flammarian, 1978); *Traditions et Soins d'aujourd'hui* (Inter Editions, 1983).

Michael MacDonald is an Associate Professor of History at the University of Wisconsin-Madison. He is the author of *Mystical Bedlam: Madness, Anxiety, and Healing in Seventeenth-Century England* (Cambridge, 1981) and a dozen articles on aspects of the social, cultural and medical history of England, 1500–1800.

Roy Porter, after taking his first degree in Cambridge, became a fellow first of Christ's College, and then of Churchill College, Cambridge, and University Lecturer in History. In 1979, he moved to the Wellcome Institute for the History of Medicine in London, where he is now Senior Lecturer in the Social History of Medicine. He has worked on the history of geology and his current work in the history of medicine focuses upon quackery, psychiatry and popular health care. He has coedited the *Dictionary of the History of Science* (Macmillan, 1981) and *The Anatomy of Madness* (2 vols., Tavistock, 1985) as well as being the author of *English Society in the Eighteenth Century* (Penguin, 1982).

Guenter B. Risse is Professor and Chairman of the Department of the History of Health Sciences, University of California at San Francisco. He holds an MD degree from the University of Buenos Aires, Argentina and a PhD from the University of Chicago. He has published on many aspects of medicine and physiology, especially on eighteenth century topics, and edited several books, including Rothschuh's *History of Physiology* (1974 and 1981) which he also translated from the German. His most recent book is *Hospital Life in Enlightenment Scotland: Care and Teaching at the Royal Infirmary of Edinburgh* (Cambridge, 1986).

Andrew Wear is Lecturer in History and Philosophy of Science at the University of Aberdeen. He has written on renaissance philosophy, medicine and anatomy and coedited *The Medical Renaissance of the Sixteenth Century* (Cambridge, 1985). His current research is on health and illness in early modern England.

E.A. Wrigley is Professor of Population Studies at the London School of Economics and an Associate Director of the Cambridge Group for the History of Population and Social Structure. He is the author of *Industrial Growth and Population Change* (1961), *Population and History* (1969) and (with Roger Schofield) *The Population History of England 1541–1871* (1981). He edited *An Introduction to English Historical Demography* (1966), *Nineteenth Century Society* (1969), *Identifying People in the Past* (1973), (with Philip Abrams) *Towns in Society* (1978), and (with David Souden) *The Works of Thomas Robert Malthus* (1986).

Acknowledgements

This book arose out of a conference held at Corpus Christi College, Cambridge in March 1985 to discuss new methods in the history of medicine.[1] The editors are extremely grateful to the Wellcome Trust for meeting the costs of that conference and for subsequently paying for the translation of papers. We would also like to thank several anonymous referees for their invaluable advice in the production of this book.

Note

1. For discussion of conference proceedings see D. Watkins, 'Problems and Methods in the History of Medicine', in the *Bulletin of the Society for the Social History of Medicine, 36* (1985), 61–4.

Introduction

Just fifteen years ago, in a collection entitled *Modern Methods in the History of Medicine*, Edwin Clarke called for the emancipation of the history of medicine from its thraldom to biobibliography and narrative.[1] It would of course be grossly misleading to infer from Clarke's rallying-call that all previous medical history had wallowed in some prehistoric 'anecdotage' — one only has to bring to mind the names of Henry Sigerist, Richard Shryock, Erwin Ackernecht, Owsei Temkin, George Rosen and many others to be made aware that the leading medical historians of a generation or two ago combined linguistic erudition and historical vision, medical expertise and cosmopolitan perspectives to a degree that can only inspire awe and envy today.[2]

Yet it is pleasant also to be able to record that the history of medicine has actually come a long way since 1971. In practically all fields covered by the contributors to Clarke's volume — the histories of public health, of hospitals, of scientific medicine and so forth — research has accelerated and intensified, thanks not least to the surging tide of Ph.D dissertations in the discipline.[3] And new sub-specialisms have emerged and gone from strength to strength where previously there were only isolated practitioners. This applies above all, perhaps, to the social history of medicine, a division that did not even warrant a separate chapter in Clarke's collection, but which now commands the allegiance of a majority of the younger scholars in the Anglo-American profession and supports a distinct institution in Britain (the Society for the Social History of Medicine, founded in 1970).

Indeed, the social history of medicine has been closely associated with a wave of radical rejection of much that traditional so-called 'Whiggish' history of medicine allegedly stood for.[4] Old-style scholarship, it has been argued, was basically 'in house', written largely by doctors about doctors for doctors, and explicitly or implicitly it sang the praises of medical progress. Many new-wave social historians of medicine have set out to 'demystify' this situation, showing that much that has passed for history has actually been covert propaganda, hagiography or ideology; and they have aimed to explore through fresh eyes, how doctors and medicine, as well as controlling disease, have also been integral to much wider, and allegedly sinister, practices of socio-political and

1

intellectual control. Neo-Marxism has directed attention to the parts played by the medical profession in the maintenance of the class system; feminist scholarship has shown how medicine perpetuates gender roles;[5] Foucault's analysis of *savoir/pouvoir* has revealed how the rise of medical intervention (traditionally regarded as a 'progressive' movement) could actually be insidiously repressive;[6] and exponents of the sociology of knowledge have convincingly demonstrated how comprehensively medical science encodes and naturalises socio-political values and programmes.[7] The age of innocence has ended.

But has it yet been replaced by an age of understanding? For many of the exciting and challenging new perspectives briefly outlined above have been programmatic and even rhetorical, sometimes relying on slogans more than scholarship. Thanks in part to partisan polemicists such as Ivan Illich,[8] many grand and illuminating phrases are reverberating around academe, notions such as social control,[9] the medicalisation of life, the policing of families,[10] the expropriation of health, and so forth — phrases that are certainly not meaningless but ones whose meaning and applicability need to be confirmed by in-depth research and critical scholarship.[11]

This is no easy task, because the fields to which such concepts apply — above all, the broad interfaces between medicine and *mentalité*, people and politics — are ones in which the data are necessarily most fragmentary and impressionistic. There may never be a final answer to the question of whether William Harvey was an Aristotelian, but the business of assembling and assessing the relevant evidence pro and con is finite. By contrast, documentary problems — problems of choice, processing, evaluation — are vastly more challenging if we are seriously to get to grips with the profound questions posed by modern perspectives in the wider, social history of medicine. Has there been an 'expropriation of health' through the development of 'medicalisation'? It is easy to suppose there has,[12] but it is impossible to be sure until we have a much clearer idea of how many professional and commercial healers there really were in pre-nineteenth century societies. Meantime, conceptual classification is needed too. For, as Colin Jones suggests in his contribution to this volume, unthinking incantation of a term like 'medicalisation' can be highly misleading. As commonly used, it evokes the imposition of hegemonic medical values and even the suppression of popular culture; but the processes involved, Jones suggests, may actually revolve around demand from below rather than domination from above.[13] Or, to take another example, was female 'hysteria' essentially a construct designed to ensure the docility and control of middle-class women, a label forced upon them by the medical profession and patriarchal society in collusion with one another? Probably, but our knowledge of the manifestations of the condition remains anecdotal and confined to certain celebrated instances. The latest research in the pipeline suggests our stereotypes may all be quite misleading: hysteria may, in reality, for instance, have been more a working class than an *haut bourgeois* manifestation.[14] Or were pre-Listerian hospitals gateways to death?[15] And if they were, then why were they founded and funded? What more oblique functions did they really fulfil? We are hardly in a position to decide, until the rich but scandalously neglected archives of the voluntary hospitals have been subjected to energetic scrutiny.[16]

Projects such as these — many more might be mentioned — open up vistas simultaneously of great opportunity but also of great difficulty. Mountains of data confront us, until now rarely systematically exploited by medical historians for what they will reveal about the health of nations, about mortality and morbidity, about past societies' experiences and encounters with sickness and suffering: materials such as baptism registers, coroners' records, the archives of charities, Poor Law disbursements, hospital admission registers, asylum casebooks, doctors' accounts, court proceedings, census returns, and not least the diaries, letters and journals of the people at large. Specialist historical demographers, legal scholars and social historians have in many cases pioneered novel and highly fruitful methods for digesting and interpreting these formidable and often intractable sources.[17] But it still largely remains up to historians of medicine, on the one hand to assimilate the work of their colleagues and enter into fruitful dialogue with them, and, on the other, to devise techniques of their own to make these documents yield up answers to the particular questions of the new historians of medicine.

It is to suchlike problems and opportunities that this book is addressed. The coherence of this collection of essays lies not in arguing a particular party line (pro or anti medical science, radical or reactionary), but in focusing on new sources, techniques, and outlooks that are currently being developed in the history of medicine and in cognate disciplines, in assessing difficulties and dividends (not in the abstract but through consideration of actual research experience), and in pointing to future prospects. Some of the most imaginative flights of theory can thereby be offered a more solid grounding.

If in the real world national boundaries have been the occasions of perennial warfare, in the academic world disciplinary boundaries perpetuate ignorance and misunderstanding. As Jean-Pierre Goubert writes in the fascinating autobiographical introduction to his contribution to this volume, his own scholarly training benefited from being situated at the heart of one of the most exciting, open-minded interdisciplinary movements of modern historical scholarship, what we may loosely call the 'Annales School', with its programmatic integration of geography and history, man and society, biology and culture. Yet, for all that, he admits his apprenticeship led him to be dismissive towards the potential insights of Freudian psycho-history, and to be deeply guarded at the arrival of Foucault's archaeological approach to human history and its structured analysis. The 'Annales School', notes Toby Gelfand in the first essay, has in many ways been remarkably receptive to medical perspectives on human history, in so far as examining the 'biology of man in history' has been made one of its goals.[18] But its labours certainly haven't integrated or bridged the outlooks of medical historians with the insights of 'total history' considered over *la longue durée*.

Far from it, in fact, for the traditional concerns of medical historians — the achievements of doctors and medical institutions, the progress of medical science, indeed the whole development of medicine over the last two centuries — have been signally absent from the pages of *Annales*. (The same strictures would apply, *mutatis mutandis*, to the ambitious programme of social history developed by such British Marxists as Rodney Hilton, Christopher Hill, E.P. Thompson and Eric Hobsbawm, and to the journal closely associated with their work, *Past and Present*.[19])

The problems of constructing histories of society and histories of medicine that do not maintain an 'armed peace' but which can interact fruitfully are tackled in several contributions to this volume. Goubert himself suggests how perhaps the most promising basis for a genuinely 'total history' lies in starting from 'total sources'. Instead of pursuing 'tunnel histories' of anatomy, midwives, medical schools or whatever, we should saturate ourselves in the entire medical experiences and activities of a particular region, developing total familiarity with the whole range of archival materials, granting no automatic privilege to 'high' (or indeed to 'popular') medicine, to official documents (or indeed, to the medical *vox populi*). It sounds one obvious solution, and it has undoubtedly been pursued with great success by French historians — though Goubert's auto-critique also lays bare some of the pitfalls of the technique.[20] Yet oddly, there has been no real equivalent at all within Anglo-Saxon scholarship. Historical medical topography seems a highly promising and entirely uncharted field.

Another area in which French scholarship has led and British research has lagged lies in the integration of medical anthropology with medical history. The explanation is perhaps simple: British medical anthropologists addressed the Empire and travelled in the bush, whereas their French equivalents still had a peasantry in their backyards. Hence an awkwardness still persists between history and anthropology amongst British academics, which, as Françoise Loux's contribution shows, is not felt amongst French connections.[21] Even Levi-Strauss's highly structuralist anthropology, when properly understood, Loux argues, is not inimical to historical thinking, and, as her own work demonstrates, abundant historical sources exist, anthropological interpretation of which will actually rescue the historian from the misunderstandings imposed by such 'historical' perspectives as evolutionary psychological positivism. Her own studies of proverbs[22] offer admirable examples of how the *mentalités* of largely pre-literate cultures have been preserved in forms relatively uncontaminated by print culture; and her discussion below of the anthropology of dirt is an object lesson in how the insights of a sister discipline can overturn some of the assumptions taken for granted by the traditional medical historian.

The problem of how to explore *mentalités* is critical to the contributions of Michael MacDonald and Andrew Wear. For MacDonald (who has written illuminatingly elsewhere of the value of anthropological approaches for the medical historian)[23] the problem is interpreting suicide. Not the traditional Durkheimian question of why people killed themselves but rather how society evaluated such acts.[24] Was it seen as a sin or a crime, an act of depression or a noble sacrifice? Did it fall within the compass of the law, the Church, or of psychological medicine? Here, Macdonald shows how one of the many series of sources hitherto underexploited by medical historians proves wonderfully helpful: coroners' rolls. These reveal two crucial dimensions. First, that different social groups commonly had distinct perceptions of the act (hence the meaning of suicide was itself the subject of conflict and negotiation). And second, that its recorded perception changed dramatically within a short space of time (secularisation). Documentary sources — evidence massive enough in scale as to require computer analysis — thus dispel ignorance and vague generalities[25] and pinpoint changes of public attitude with surprising exactitude.

Of course, the computer doesn't then interpret for us the meaning of these shifts. And so both MacDonald and Wear (in his own exploration of the problems of unravelling early modern sickness experiences)[26] therefore take up the problem of how to superimpose and integrate distinctive sorts of evidence, above all, the quantitative and qualitative.

The historian who keeps faith with traditional qualitative methods — scanning texts, picking up 'impressions' from them, illustrating them with quotations — may well seem to be (as Keith Thomas has noted) an academic throw-back wielding his bow and arrow in a nuclear age. Yet, as MacDonald argues, frank subjectivity is wholly preferable to the spurious 'objectivity' that comes of cavalierly reducing the polyvalent phrases of historical documents to machine-readable symbols, eliminating nuance in the drive for numbers. Cultural historians must indeed learn to count, but even so, semiotics is not statistics. Both have their place, but making valid translations between them remains immensely difficult. As MacDonald points out, when some years ago he was confronted with some thousands of casenotes and diagnoses in the manuscripts of the early-seventeenth-century physician, Richard Napier,[27] the range of analytical operations that computer programmes could then usefully perform on them, without involving gross over-simplification, was quite limited. Things are, however, changing and some of the newer possibilities of what more sophisticated programmes can achieve through content analysis of essentially qualitative data are mentioned by MacDonald.

The rise of computing is not the only 'new method' in the history of medicine not prophesied in Clarke's 1971 book; but it would be hard to deny that its adoption seems set fair to transform the practice of history more than any comparable innovation since the great 'opening of the archives' of the nineteenth century — though Le Roy Ladurie's prediction that the non-computerised historian would rapidly become a dinosaur seems to under-rate the conservative tenacity of the profession.[28] It is right to be wary of the cult of the computers. But it is more important to explore and refine what they can achieve. Two chapters in this volume, those by Guenter Risse and by Anne Digby, do just that, describing and evaluating strategies that they themselves adopted in research projects for which the availability of the computer has made in-depth analysis possible to a degree that proved far too daunting to scholars in the pre-computer age.

It has long been known that the Edinburgh Infirmary possesses extraordinarily fine records, admission registers and especially patient case histories; but the very richness of this kind of material has paradoxically hitherto hindered rather than forwarded the idea of constructing histories that centred on the patient as the focus of a hospital's activities.[29] What sort and class of patient was principally admitted? What were the characteristic complaints from which they were suffering? How were they treated? How long did they stay? How many recovered? How many died? Most hospital histories hitherto have typically ducked such questions, given a few juicy extracts out of minute books, or simply repeated data out of annual reports or printed rules. By putting a computer to work Risse demonstrates that we can obtain a statistical profile of the Infirmary that tears off many of the veils of the impressionistic and the ideological; and in so doing, he has shown how hospital records can thenceforth profitably be used as major indices not just of hospital practice but of community health and sickness.[30]

If hospital accounts have been dogged with ignorance and prejudice, how much more does that judgement apply to asylum histories. Emotive images of these ('museums of madness')[31] litter the pages of histories of psychiatry almost in inverse proportion to our ignorance of their operation. Yet for many mental hospitals, impressive records do actually survive, and Digby demonstrates, in her account of the strategies she adopted in her computer-based study of the York Retreat, how sensitive programming and careful evaluation of print-outs can modify the most ingrained stereotypes, and open up new questions for research.[32] Did, for example, the Victorian asylum 'silt up' with patients who, once admitted, never got out? A superficial glance at the figures seems to confirm this emotive stereotype. Sophisticated computer analysis, however, shows that the great majority of patients remained short-stay, and that a small core of chronic cases all too readily distorts the picture.

Qualitative and quantitative evidence must ultimately mesh because both relate to the same objects: people. The artificial sub-divisions of the historical profession all too readily result in treating human beings rather as Cartesian divided selves, a biological animal scrutinised by historical demographers on the one hand, thumbing through their life-tables of births, marriages and deaths, and on the other, a cultural being, interpreted by socio-intellectual historians. But such hard-and-fast distinctions are utterly false, and one of the major aims of the two papers in this collection by historical demographers, Tony Wrigley and Arthur Imhof, is to remind us all of the ultimate unity of the biological and cultural. 'Biological' events — birth-rates, population aggregates — are of course determined by biological variables — by disease, death, and nutritional levels, by micro-organisms and vitamins; but these themselves operate only in a complex dialectic with cultural choices: the social distribution of natural resources, customary patterns of marriage, and so forth. As Wrigley argues, fluctuations in population bear witness to myriad social choices (along a continuum from the planned to the unconscious) no less than to the bacteria. Thus the North-West European pattern of late marriage is inseparable from a society whose biological death-rate is not calamitously high. And in turn (as emerges from the climax of Imhof's paper), the facts of 'birth, copulation, and death' also shape consciousness. Perhaps the 'sudden death' biology of the world of the subsistence crisis produced the *mentalité* of the eternal life in heaven.

This book does not map out 'five-year plans' for future research, not least because it is futile to abstract methods from matter: methods are not universal but advance through the needs and opportunities of particular materials. Hence the focus here has been to present reflections by leading historians on techniques and perspectives developed by them within specific research contexts but hopefully relevant to the situations of fellow researchers. We look to a future medical history that will benefit more fully from advances in parallel fields of inquiry and make its own fuller contributions to them as well. We trust this volume will prove some stimulus in that direction.

Notes

1. E. Clarke (ed.), *Modern Methods in the History of Medicine* (London: Athlone Press, 1971).
2. For valuable perspectives on the development of the history of

medicine see Charles Webster, 'The Historiography of Medicine', in P. Corsi and P. Weindling (eds.), *Information Sources in the History of Science and Medicine* (London, Butterworth, 1983), 29–43.

3. Much of this work is listed and discussed in Margaret Pelling, 'Medicine since 1500', in Corsi and Weindling (eds.), *Information Sources*, 379–410, and Gert H. Brieger, 'History and Medicine', in P.T. Durbin (ed.), *A Guide to the Culture of Science, Technology and Medicine* (New York, Collier Macmillan, 1980), 121–96.

4. For discussion of the new social history of medicine see P. Wright and A. Treacher (eds.), *The Problem of Medical Knowledge* (Edinburgh, 1982); J. Woodward and D. Richards (eds.), 'Towards a Social History of Medicine', in *Health Care and Popular Medicine in Nineteenth Century England* (London, Croom Helm, 1977), 15–55. See also L.J. Jordanova, 'The Social Sciences and History of Science and Medicine', in Corsi and Weindling (eds.), *Information Sources,* 81–98.

5. For a broad survey see Y. Knibiehler and C. Fouquet, *La Femme et Les Médecins. Analyse Historique* (Paris, Hachette, 1983). See also J. Leavitt (ed.), *Women and Health in America* (Madison, University of Wisconsin Press, 1984), and for an assessment of Marxism, Karl Figlio, 'Sinister Medicine? A Critique of Left Approaches to Medicine', *Radical Science Journal, 9* (1979), 14–68.

6. See M. Foucault, *Histoire de la Folie à l'âge Classique* (Paris, 1961). Translated as *Madness and Civilization* (New York, Mentor, 1965); *idem, The Order of Things* (New York, Vintage Books, 1973); *idem, The Birth of the Clinic,* trans. A.M. Sheridan Smith (New York, Vintage Books, 1975); *idem, The Archeology of Knowledge,* trans. A.M. Sheridan Smith (London, Tavistock, 1972).

7. See Jordanova, in Corsi and Weindling (eds.), *Information Sources,* 81–98.

8. See especially I. Illich, *Limits to Medicine* (Harmondsworth, Penguin, 1963).

9. For an evaluation of the use of this concept see S. Cohen and A. Scull (eds.), *Social Control and the State* (Oxford, Basil Blackwell, 1983).

10. See J. Donzelot, *The Policing of Families* (London, Hutchinson, 1980).

11. For example, the scholarly basis of much of Foucault's work has come under fire. See H.C. Erik Midelfort, 'Madness and Civilization in Early Modern Europe', in Barbara Malament (ed.), *After the Reformation* (Philadelphia, University of Pennsylvania Press, 1980); Lawrence Stone, 'Madness', *The New York Review of Books, 29* (16 December 1982), 28–30.

12. For scholarship within the 'medicalisation' mould see P. Goubert (ed.), *La Médicalisation de la Société Française 1770–1830* (Waterloo, Ontario, 1982).

13. There is an interesting discussion of 'medical consumerism' in H. Cook, *The Decline of the Old Medical Regime in Stuart London* (Ithaca, Cornell University Press, 1986). See also, C. Lawrence, 'William Buchan: Medicine Laid Open', *Medical History, 19* (1975), 20–35.

14. See Edward Shorter, 'Paralysis: The Rise and Fall of a "Hysterical" Symptom', *Journal of Social History, 19* (1986), 549–82. For traditional history of hysteria, see I. Vieth, *Hysteria* (Chicago, University

Press, 1945); for a feminist perspective see D. Ehrenreich and B. English, *For Her Own Good. 150 Years of the Experts Advice to Women* (London, Pluto Press, 1979).

15. See T. McKeown and R.G. Brown, 'Medical Evidence Related to English Population Changes in the Eighteenth Century', *Population Studies, 9* (1955–6), 119–41: for a subsequent opinion see S. Cherry, 'The Hospitals and Population Growth: the Voluntary General Hospitals, Mortality and Local Populations in the English Provinces in the Eighteenth and Nineteenth Centuries', *Population Studies, 34* (1980), 59–75, 251–65.

16. For discussion of the salubrity of hospitals, see J. Woodward, *To Do the Sick No Harm. A Study of the British Voluntary Hospital System to 1875* (London, Routledge and Kegan Paul, 1974).

17. E.g., for historical demography see E.A. Wrigley and R. Schofield, *The Population History of England. A Reconstitution* (London, Edward Arnold, 1981); or for legal records, R.F. Hunnisett, *The Medieval Coroner* (Cambridge, University Press, 1961); *idem* (ed.), *Calendar of Nottinghamshire Coroners Inquests, Thoroton Society Record Series, 25* (Nottingham, 1969); *idem*, 'The Importance of Eighteenth Century Coroners' Bills' in E.W. Ives and A.H. Manchester (eds.), *Law, Litigants, and the Legal Profession* (London, Royal Historical Society, 1983).

18. For further analysis of *Annaliste* history, see Peter Burke, 'Revolution in Popular Culture', in Roy Porter and Mikuláš Teich (eds.), *Revolution in History* (Cambridge, University Press, 1986), 206–25. For an instance see Jean-Pierre Peter, 'Maladies à la Fin du XVIIIe Siècle', *Annales: E.S.C., 22* (1967), 711–51. Some *Annales* articles dealing with medical topics are usefully translated in R. Forster and O. Ranum (eds.), *Biology of Man in History. Selections from the Annales,* trans. by E. Forster and P.M. Ranum (Baltimore, Johns Hopkins University Press, 1975).

19. Harvey J. Kaye, *The British Marxist Historians* (Cambridge, Polity Press, 1984). Of course, some valuable contributions have appeared in *Past and Present*. See for example Patricia Crawford, 'Attitudes to Menstruation in Seventeenth-Century England', *Past and Present, 91* (1981), 47–73.

20. See of course Goubert's own *Malades et Médecine en Bretagne 1770–1790* (Paris, 1974), and also Alain Croix, *La Bretagne aux 16e et 17e Siècles. La Vie-La Mort-La Foi,* 2 Vols. (Paris, 1981).

21. For an admirable discussion see Michael MacDonald, 'Anthropological Perspectives on the History of Science and Medicine', in Corsi and Weindling (eds.), *Information Sources,* 61–80. See also, Carlo Ginzburg, 'Anthropology and History in the 1980s. A Comment', in T. Rabb and R.I. Rotberg, *The New History, the 1980s and Beyond* (Princeton, 1982).

22. Françoise Loux, *Le Corps Dans la Société Traditionnelle* (Paris, Berger-Levrault, 1979), and Françoise Loux and Philippe Richard, *Sagesses du Corps, Santé et Maladie dans les Proverbs Regionaux Françaises* (Paris, Maisonneuve et Larose, 1978). Proverbs have received far less attention from English-speaking scholars, though see J. Obelkevitch, 'Proverbs and Social History', in P. Burke and R. Porter (eds.), *The Social History of Language* (Cambridge, University Press, 1987). For another instance of the successful use of anthropological perspectives see J. Gelis, *L'arbre et le*

Fruit. La Naissance dans l'Occident Moderne XVIe–XIXe Siècle (Paris, Fayard, 1984).

23. MacDonald, in Corsi and Weindling (eds.), *Information Sources,* 61–80.

24. See also Michael MacDonald, 'The Inner Side of Wisdom: Suicide in Early Modern England', *Psychological Medicine, 7* (1977), 565–83; *idem,* 'The Secularization of Suicide in England 1660–1800', *Past and Present,* no. 111 (1986), 50–100.

25. For such literary specialisations see S.E. Sprott, *The English Debate on Suicide* (La Salle, Ill., Open Court, 1961); Lester Crocker, 'The Discussion of Suicide in the Eighteenth Century' *Journal of the History of Ideas, 13* (1952), 47–59.

26. A discussion that amplifies some of the issues broached in his 'Puritan Perceptions of Illness in Seventeenth Century England', in Roy Porter (ed.), *Patients and Practitioners: Lay Perceptions of Medicine in Pre-Industrial England* (Cambridge, University Press, 1985), 55–100.

27. Michael MacDonald, *Mystical Bedlam* (Cambridge, University Press, 1981).

28. See Roderick Floud, 'Quantitative History and People's History. Two Methods in Conflict', *Social Science History, 8* (1984), 151–68. See also the journal, *Historical Methods.* Quantification and computerisation as historical methods came of age for English historians with the foundation of The Association for History and Computing during 1986. At its inaugural conference (March 21st–23rd) over forty papers were presented covering topics ranging from the analysis of regional settlement in ancient Greece to the uses of the computer made by economic historians of modernity. Small studies such as W. Vaughan's 'Computers and Pictorial Analysis. The Automated Connoisseur', were illustrated, together with very large projects such as the computerisation of the Domesday Book, presented by a team from Hull University, John Palmer, Andrew Ayton and Virginia Davies; see 'History and Computing', *The Inaugural Conference of the Association for History and Computing* (Institute of Historical Research, 1986).

29. See more broadly Roy Porter, 'The Patient's View: Doing History from Below', *Theory and Society, 14* (1985), 175–98.

30. See for the fuller study G. Risse, *Hospital Life in Enlightenment Scotland. Care and Teaching at the Royal Infirmary of Edinburgh* (Cambridge, University Press, 1986). It should be compared with the standard history, A. Logan Turner, *Story of a Great Hospital: The Royal Infirmary of Edinburgh 1729–1929* (Edinburgh, Oliver and Boyd, 1937).

31. See A.T. Scull, *Museums of Madness: the Social Organisation of Insanity in Nineteenth-Century England* (London, Allen Lane, 1979); *idem* (ed.), *Madhouses, Mad-Doctors, and Madmen* (Philadelphia, University of Pennsylvania Press, 1981).

32. For wider study, see Anne Digby, *Madness, Morality and Medicine* (Cambridge, University Press, 1985).

I

The French Connection

1

The *Annales* and Medical Historiography: *Bilan et Perspectives**

Toby Gelfand

The influence of the movement in French historiography known as the *Annales* school upon medical historians has been incalculable. Incalculable in importance because, like all historians concerned to situate their particular domain in the broadest possible framework, medical historians have increasingly in recent decades sought to connect health, disease and medicine with other structures in societies of the past. The syncretic application of theory, method, and data from the entire spectrum of social and behavioural sciences to history, pioneered by the *Annales* as *histoire totale*, has been a major historiographical development of the second third of our century.[1] Practitioners of the so-called new social history of medicine, whether in Britain, North America, Germany or elsewhere, have profited from the *Annales* precedent, even if their debt is most often indirect and not easily demonstrable. Needless to say, the connection is most easily visible in medical history written by the French and by those in other countries who work on the history of French medicine.[2] In some measure, however, social historians of medicine everywhere are Annalistes.

The problem, of course, is determining that 'measure'. How can one measure an influence that appears pervasive and yet notoriously difficult to pin down, much less calculate? Lucien Febvre, a founding father of the *Annales*, cautioned against the epistemological weakness of the notion of historical 'influence'. Febvre suggested the elimination of the mysterious astrological

---

* Revised version of paper read at the Conference on Problems and Methods in the History of Medicine, Corpus Christi College, Cambridge University, England, March, 1985.

term in favour of 'rapport' or relations.[3] Assuming the rapport of the *Annales* with medical history writing still leaves the problem of defining the *Annales*. Febvre's successor, Fernand Braudel, thought the *Annales* had become 'a sort of intellectual epidemic'.[4] Jacques Revel, one of Braudel's current successors, has spoken of 'a movement, a sensitivity, strategies, an activity with little regard deep down for theoretical definitions.' Noting that a history of the *Annales* movement remains to be written, Revel rejects interpretations that have assumed the existence of an *Annales* 'school' or special interest group, endowed with a monolithic ideology or methodology.[5]

Nevertheless, a few things are clear. The *Annales* was and is a learned journal founded in 1929 by two professors then at the University of Strasbourg, Lucien Febvre and Marc Bloch. In terms of chronological development, most agree there have been at least three or four *Annales*: the Febvre–Bloch decade leading up to the war during which the journal bore the title *Annales d'Histoire Economique et Sociale*; the Febvre *Annales*: *Economies, Sociétés, Civilisations,* ending with the founder's death in 1956; the Braudel *Annales*, ending in the late sixties; and the post-Braudelian ongoing period in which editorial responsibility has been shared among several, including Jacques LeGoff, Emmanuel Le Roy Ladurie, Marc Ferro, Revel, and others. In schematic fashion, the leitmotifs have been successively as follows: (1) economic and social history (reflected in the original title of the review), (2) the history of quasi-permanent or very slowly changing material structures — the underlying geographical, climatological, biological, demographic, and technological determinants that shaped very broad, if not global, societies over long time periods (in Braudel's phrase, the study of the *longue durée*), and (3) an interest in the historical investigation of local systems of collective belief and behaviour susceptible to anthropological and ethnological methods of analysis.

Rather than attempting to pursue logical connections between the *Annales*' programmatic interests, as just sketched, and medical history as currently practised — this would be an enormous and highly problematic job — I shall instead look at what the *Annales* has in fact published in medical history. This straight-forward, admittedly simplistic approach may reveal more about the influence of medical history upon the *Annales* than vice versa, but it has the distinct advantage of providing us with concrete achievements (what Erwin Ackerknecht called in another context a 'behaviorist approach' to medical historiography).[6] In keeping with Revel's point, the *Annales* should be assessed in terms of what it has done, not, as has perhaps too often been the case, against some supposed paradigm.

There are several legitimate objections to inventorying (perhaps auscultating would be more apt) the *Annales* for medical historical articles.

First, it is obvious that a considerable amount of medical history informed by Annaliste ways of thinking has been published outside the pages of the 'mother' review. Individual articles, collections within and even the dedication of entire numbers of historical journals not ordinarily concerned with history of medicine bear witness to the diffusion of 'medical history *Annales* style' into general historical reviews. Examples over the past decade are: *Ethnologie Française* (nos. 3–4, 1976), *Journal of Social History* (no. 4, 1977), *Annales de Bretagne* (no. 3, 1979), *Revue d'Histoire Moderne et Contemporaine* (July-Sept. 1980), and *Reflexions Historiques—Historical Reflections* (1982). There have also been collections like *Médecins, climat et épidémies à la fin du XVIIIe siècle* (published by the VIe section of the Ecole Pratique des Hautes Études, 1972), and several volumes edited by Arthur E. Imhof, beginning with *Mensch und Gesundheit in der Geschichte* (1980). Finally, monographs written by French scholars François Lebrun, Jean-Pierre Goubert, Jacques Léonard, Jean-Noel Biraben, Françoise Loux, Vincent-Pierre Comiti, Mireille Laget, Marie-Christine Pouchelle, Jacques Gélis and others provide copious evidence of *Annales'* 'influence'.[7]

Most of these people have also published in the *Annales* and thus their work will not be wholly ignored here. But by limiting our survey to the *Annales* itself, a good deal of *Annales*-inspired medical historiography inevitably gets left out.

Second, the *Annales*, whatever its tacit party-line may have been, did not adhere to any inflexible editorial policy. There has always been a degree of pluralism in the acceptance of articles for publication. Thus the *Annales* has contained work on the history of medicine that does not otherwise look like the work of Annalistes. This paradox results from an openness to other French historiographical perspectives as well as to those of diverse foreign authors. Examples will be cited later when I sum up the pattern of *Annales* contributions to medical historiography.

Third, and most problematic, is whether the *Annales* can be said to take an interest in medical history *per se*. From the outset of the enterprise, Lucien Febvre stubbornly combatted the tendency he perceived toward specialisation along disciplinary lines. Cultivating narrow historiographical gardens might be essential to scholarship, but the garden walls, Febvre argued, threatened to hide work in one plot from others to which it was intimately connected.[8]

For Febvre, historical problems, problems of societies, did not respect disciplinary boundaries. When asked by a geographer where geography would appear in a multi-volume inter-disciplinary encyclopaedia he was planning, Febvre, who had truly encyclopaedic knowledge and interests, replied: 'why, my dear colleague, everywhere and nowhere'.[9] The same was true for history of art, the law, morality and so on. Clearly, Febvre's 'everywhere and nowhere' answer applied to science and medicine too. By and large, the *Annales* has kept faith with anti-specialisation as formulated in the quest toward an all-embracing concept of *histoire totale*. Despite the fact that since the late 1960s, for a variety of reasons, not the least of which has been the *tour de force* of Michel Foucault, the emphasis has shifted from global aspirations à la Febvre and Braudel to local or micro studies, the multi-disciplinary ideal remains.

The possibility of medical history being 'everywhere and nowhere' in the *Annales* presents an undeniable practical problem for our survey. I have not attempted to read every article published since 1929. It is entirely possible, indeed probable, that descriptive data and analytical aperçus relevant to medical history are dissolved into the fabric of *Annales* articles the titles of which give little hint of their presence. It is also likely that articles on demography, as is the case with the demographic sections of most *Annales*-inspired doctoral theses on regions of France (e.g. those by Pierre Goubert, Georges Frêche, Jean-Claude Perrot) contain discussions of epidemic diseases, hospitals, medical personnel, etc.[10]

Conversely one might conceivably argue that some of the *Annales* articles I have designated as medical historical are really some other kind of history. Virtually all the authors would, if asked, probably eschew the professional label of medical historian in favour of a rubric more in the mainstream of historiography.

This problem of categorising obviously becomes more acute as one attempts to break down medical history into sub-themes. In the end, my effort at classification, like all taxonomies, must be seen as artificial, arbitrary, and tentative, a heuristic approach whose only proof, like puddings, is in the tasting.

Keeping the above qualifications in mind, let us turn to the data. I have designated as medical historical a total of 55 articles published in the *Annales*, 17 of which appeared in two special numbers. These will be considered as two separate though obviously connected groups of 38 and 17 contributions.

First, a chronological analysis by decade of publications on medical history (see Figure 1.1) shows but a single article during the first 20 years of the *Annales*. Between 1950 and 1959, one finds three articles. Then during the 1960s there is a striking increase — eight publications on medical history and a special number at the end of the decade, *Histoire biologique et société*, with seven contributions on medical history. The 1970s brought an acceleration of the trend, a doubling — 15 articles and a second special number, in September-October 1977, this time devoted entirely to ten articles under the title *Médecins, Médecine et Société en France aux XVIIIe et XIXe siècles*. It would be premature to say whether the pace will continue in the 1980s but there is evidence of a decline, or at least a leveling off, with six publications to date through the first half of the decade.

In summary, the *Annales* output in medical history, although modest quantitatively (probably of the order of 1 to 3 per cent of the articles), is perceptible and shows a definite pattern of development.[11] The near absence during the Febvre-Bloch years is, at first glance, somewhat surprising, given Bloch's brilliant precedent in his early masterpiece on the royal healing touch for scrofula, *Les Rois Thaumaturges* (1924), and Febvre's broadly conceived bio-geographical, *La Terre et l'évolution humaine* (1922). Febvre, moreover, displayed genuine empathy for 'neglected neighbors or brothers' among whom he counted historians of science.[12] None the less, during the inter-war decades such disciplines remained marginal to the historical enterprise and, in general, poorly professionalised, despite heroic efforts by scholars like George Sarton and Henry Sigerist, two émigré Europeans (a Belgian and Swiss) who became founding figures within American universities for history of science and history of medicine, respectively.[13]

In France, practitioners of these fields tended to be academic scientists, physicians, or philosophers whose contributions usually appeared in specialised journals dependent upon the parent discipline. Even Febvre acknowledged such cleavages. In 1927, reviewing a study on biological thought in the 18th and early 19th

Figure 1.1: Annales *publications in history of medicine (by decade). Hatched area represents special numbers*

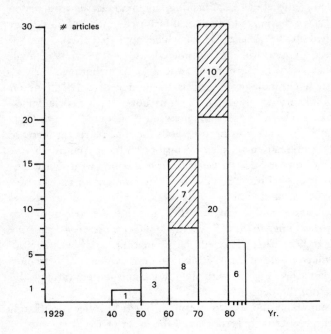

centuries, Febvre called for a 'social history of scientific ideas'. The time had not yet come, however, he remarked, when ordinary historians could undertake this new task. It would have to be left to specialists with expert knowledge.[14] In this spirit, the Febvre-Bloch *Annales*, often Febvre personally, reviewed books on medical history written by medical doctors.[15]

In 1947, a professor on the medical faculty at Strasbourg University wrote the *Annales'* first medical historical article, a discussion of the decline of malaria in France. Although a modest, even humble, beginning (Dr Callot feared his eight-page essay had been too long), this first contribution foreshadowed in significant ways the *Annales'* later approach to medical history. The author presented a critical review of the problems of retrospective diagnosis of the disease, its clinical course, epidemiology and the natural history of the vector. Underlying the biological and demographic perspective was the suggestion that human factors, such as changes in the peasant economy, were most pertinent to the problem of the decline of malaria.[16]

In the 1960s, after an interval of more than a decade, the *Annales*, under the aegis of Fernand Braudel, took up, this time in a systematic and sustained way, an inquiry into bio-medical aspects of history. In 1961, four years after he succeeded Febvre as chief director of the *Annales*, Braudel launched an *enquête* into 'the history of material life and biological patterns of behavior'.[17] Braudel candidly explained that his own research interests formed the point of departure for the new endeavour, interests reflected in his thesis, *La Méditerranée et le monde Méditerranéen à l'époque de Philippe II* (1949), and which would reach a culmination in his three-volume *Civilisation matérielle et Capitalisme (XVe–XVIIIe siècle)* (1967, 1979). Braudel's ambitious *enquête* on material life extended an open invitation to historians and non-historians to contribute new perspectives from 'geography, anthropology, sociology, economics, demography, folklore, prehistory, linguistics, medicine, statistics . . .'.[18]

Over the following three years, *Annales*' publications on biology and medicine included two short notices by Jean-Paul Aron on biology and alimentation (1961) and the reciprocal interactions of biology and history (1962), two articles on the black death of the 14th century, the one a lengthy study of famines and epidemics by Elisabeth Carpentier (1962), the other a brief remark on the black death in Bohemia by F. Grause (1963), and an essay on historical pathology by Mirko Grmek (1963).

In 1966, the *Annales* published its first report on a new and much more specific medical historical *enquête* led by Jean Meyer and Le Roy Ladurie under the auspices of the VIe section of the Ecole Pratique des Hautes Etudes (EPHE). Meyer's article introduced and brought widespread attention to the previously neglected archives of the Paris Société Royale de Médecine dating from the final 20 years of the Old Regime. These vast archives containing doctor's reports on epidemic diseases represented an historical gold mine awaiting exploration and exploitation, and they have since served as a major source for *Annales* medical history.

Jean-Pierre Peter quickly followed Meyer's publication with a second article on the Société Royale archives. Peter's 'Malades et maladies à la fin du XVIIIe siècle' (1967), although presented as a preliminary report — 'un premier aperçu' — was in fact an extensive and subtle analysis running to 40 pages, the longest article on medical history in the *Annales*. I shall later argue that it was also a seminal work for *Annales* medical historiography since

21

Peter attempted from within the now-familiar context of Braudel's emphasis on the history of material life to introduce a new dimension.

The decade of the 60s, the decade of the Braudelian *Annales*, closed with a special number devoted to biological history and society that faithfully mirrored the programme launched by Braudel at the outset of the period. Of the seven contributions dealing with disease (two other sections of the number took up demography and alimentation), five were heavily epidemiological in orientation: Biraben and LeGoff's extensive inventory of bubonic plague in the early middle ages, Vincent on plagues in the kingdom of Grenada in the 16th and 17th centuries, Valensi on demographic calamities in Tunisia and in the eastern Mediterranean in the 18th and 19th centuries, Jean-Pierre Goubert on epidemics in Brittany at the end of the 18th century, and Le Roy Ladurie's review of famine amenorrhoea from the 17th to the 20th century. Only two articles departed from retrospective demography as a way of understanding disease: Grmek proposed theoretical frameworks for looking at disease in history and Sigal discussed miracle cures at Reims.

At this juncture it should be obvious that Fernand Braudel had imposed his stamp upon *Annales* medical history as indeed upon much else published in the journal during the late 1950s and 1960s. In their unsigned preface to the special number of 1969, the new editors hastened to reassure readers that the *Annales* had not become converted to an exclusive concern with 'the opaque problems of the sub-basement of human history, to the part which is least dynamic, voluntary, and human'. They insisted rather that the emphasis on biological history sought to redress an imbalance created by a scholastic separation of the history of the body from the spirit; the new editors reaffirmed their fidelity to the credo of the founders, Bloch and Febvre, that history should be about man, or better, about men.[19]

One is tempted to comment that the '*Annales* doth protest too much'. Under the leadership of Braudel, the journal had displayed little interest in individual historical actors or small communities; people tended to be analysed as populations shaped by static structures over which they had little control or understanding. Braudel's *longue durée*, a concept formally propounded in an essay in the 'Débats et Combats' section of the *Annales* in 1958, favoured historical time units measured in centuries, units longer than any human lifetime.

As is well known, the *longue durée* paradigm, concretely embodied in Braudel's thesis on the Mediterranean, implied a history of society built upon the physical and biological bedrock of climate, geography, geology, demography, physical anthropology and material culture. Only after this structure had been defined could one properly situate economic history at the centre of the Braudelian project. Neglected or scarcely attained by this approach were the upper reaches of the total history envisaged, encouraged and practised by Febvre and Bloch — the history of *mentalité* or popular culture as well as the history of high culture or intellectual history on which historians of science and medicine traditionally laboured.[20]

During the 1960s, publications in the *Annales* incorporated biology and various specialised medical sciences such as epidemiology, pathology and haematology into their analytical framework. These fields were used for the most part methodologically and technically in order to provide more powerful explanations of demographic and especially epidemic patterns. If valuable insights were achieved, this approach failed to recognise the problems inherent in viewing biology and medicine simply as technical historical tools. Beyond the epistemological pitfalls of plugging modern sciences into fragmentary data from mediaeval and early modern sources, there was a failure to appreciate a crucial distinction between medicine in history and the history of medicine and the difficulties of applying the first without understanding the second. While medicine in history was used as a technique, the history of medicine's complex changing development as an enterprise, arising out of theoretical discourse, professional interests, institutional resources and practices, were largely left aside.

This orientation reflected, as I have already suggested, the deliberate editorial policy of the Braudel-led *Annales*. It crystallised in the 1960s and had not been characteristic of the three *Annales* publications on medical history in the prior decade: René Baehrel on class hatred during epidemics (1952; a study of mentalité that Febvre had singled out for praise), Mazaheri on Paracelsus as alchemist (1956), and Ehrard on medical ideas about plague and contagion in 18th-century France (1957).

Did the pattern of *Annales* medical historiography established in the 1960s then continue during the following decades down to the present? Before addressing this question, I want to turn to a quite different historiographical development that had a decisive impact on certain Annalistes (and many other historians as well). The work of Michel Foucault, whose *Histoire de la Folie* (1961) and *Naissance de la Clinique* (1963) in particular dealt with the history of medicine, made its presence felt in the pages of the *Annales* before the end of the 1960s.

I shall not attempt the daunting task of summarising the remarkable oeuvre of Foucault nor its relationship with what Marc Bloch called the 'historian's craft.'[21] Suffice it to note that Foucault's attention to epistemology, his penchant for a Nietzschean reading of texts, and, as a student of Georges Canguilhem, his impressive knowledge of the history and philosophy of the life sciences and psychopathology, gave him a quite different perspective from the professedly atheoretical, data-collecting, and, at times, frankly positivistic historians of the *Annales* persuasion.

Given Foucault's enormous importance and ever-augmenting stature on the French intellectual scene for the two decades prior to his death in 1984, it is not surprising that spokesmen for the *Annales* sought from time to time to reconcile his work with their own.[22] During his lifetime, the contrasts between Foucault and *Annales* history were striking; Foucault's assumption of historical discontinuities or epistemological mutations, his analysis of scientific and other specialised disciplinary discourses, his location of political and social power in what seemed to be marginal institutions like the hospital or the prison, his emotive literary language rich in metaphor and metaphysical flights, his indifference to quantitative methods and his often blatant disregard for the standard canons of selection and criticism of historical sources, all distanced Foucault from the *Annales* of Fernand Braudel.

Just a few months before Foucault's death, the historian Arlette Farge characterised his relationship with historians as a 'no man's land' and an 'espace blanc'.[23] Yet Farge, who writes on the history of popular culture (and contributed an article on occupational diseases of artisans to the *Annales* special number on medical history) herself collaborated with Foucault. If Foucault disclaimed any affiliation with historians, including the Annalistes, the latter have sought to assimilate his work. Braudel himself referred to Foucault as 'the only successor' to Lucien Febvre on the terrain of cultural history while, at the same time, deploring his lack of historical training and his tendency to be 'trop événementialiste'.[24]

Foucault's book on madness received an enthusiastic review

from Robert Mandrou in the *Annales* in 1962.[25] But not until 1967 did Jean-Pierre Peter present to *Annales* readers an alternative framework for research in medical history, an alternative to the Braudelian concept of medical history as simply a means for reconstructing material life. Peter's *démarche*, I think, can be attributed in part to Foucault's inspiration. Although he mentioned Foucault explicitly only in passing — in distinguishing the achievement of a 'geology of medical thought' in *Naissance de la Clinique* from an 'archeology of disease', the task Peter had embarked upon with the archives of the Société Royale de Médecine — Peter's deeper affinity to the Foucaultian agenda can be discerned.[26]

For one thing, Peter did not entirely succeed in doing 'archeology of disease' rather than 'geology of medical thought'; his article in fact contains quite a bit of each. The archaeology metaphor itself derived from Foucault, who had subtitled his book on the clinic an 'archéologie du régard médical' and his major work *Les mots et les choses: une archéologie des sciences humains* (1966).[27]

One can read Peter's essay on two levels. On the surface it falls comfortably within the Braudelian framework and is even compatible with an older internal medical historiographical tradition of seeking to make retrospective diagnoses. Peter, a junior member of a research *équipe*, was ostensibly submitting preliminary findings of a continuing *enquête* on epidemic diseases in France at the end of the 18th century. He sketches the protocol for a rigorous quantitative analysis of a huge archive in series consisting of hundreds of doctors' monthly reports over several decades. He outlines how he will decode 18th-century nosology, translating the old disease names when possible into modern equivalents. By means of a few illustrative cases, he graciously spares the reader a detailed immersion into the data pool of 420 disease entities and syndromes in localities scattered throughout France, data that he has collected on 3500 cards, coded and readied for the computer. Peter's approach then at this level is resolutely empirical and positivist; he is confident that the names of diseases can be translated and his concern is straightforward epidemiology:

> Our work will be concerned with disease rather than with the sick person. It will not worry about the individual, at least not as a demographic unit. We will find out which

diseases were endemic and which were receding; we will know which of them raged locally and which, on the contrary, blazed a fiery trail; we will be able to find clusters, cycles, isolated outbreaks, and tidal waves.[28]

On a second, deeper level, however, Peter presents a rather different set of attitudes and concerns. Belying the image of the dispassionate data collector, he employs a literary style suffused with emotion, struggle, and a sense of adventure evident in his opening line: 'Qui voudrait faire un voyage fantastique, celui-ci ira plonger dans les archives anciennes de la Société Royale de Médecine.' Moreover, Peter is unable to avoid the geology of medical thought or as we might say the history of medical ideas. In substance and style echoing Foucault, he writes:

Le corps de documents formé par les réponses à l'enquête de la Société Royale témoigne d'un moment privilégié dans l'histoire de la médecine. La pensée médicale s'y montre en gésine; inconsciente d'ailleurs de sa propre aventure. Ce qu'on y sent mûrir, c'est une nouvelle intelligence des rapports de la vie et de la maladie. Le médecin, placé au confluent de l'une et de l'autre, ressent que son action est appelée à changer et de sens et de terrain. Il entrevoit pour la première fois, au-delà des chimères de doctrine qui le lui cachent encore, l'objet de son effort: la maladie logée, inscrite dans le corps, dans l'homme. Jusqu'alors, elle existait pour soi, en soi. L'organisme malade, peu à peu, émerge à la conscience, à la vue.[29]

Again, sounding a Foucaultian hermeneutic note mixed with some old-fashioned Whig history of ideas, Peter speaks of medicine on the eve of the French Revolution 'forcing the locks of its theoretical prison [in which] all the work of Bichat and Laennec was already potentially there . . .'[30]

Finally, in the concluding section entitled 'morbidité et société', Peter abandons all pretence of epidemiology in order to let his archives sing their 'song' of human misery. He situates epidemic physicians' perceptions of the poor in an ethnological framework of contrasting cultures and relations of power; he speculates that numerous accounts of convulsions, especially among women, might signify an inarticulate somatic protest, a 'profound hysteroid tendency characteristic of the society of the

Old Regime, at least among the common people.'[31] Here we have come full circle back to epidemics, but we are a long way indeed from the empirical, quantitative, material-life framework with which Peter began as a faithful disciple of the Braudelian *Annales*.

I have discussed the Peter article at length because it testifies to, and perhaps crystallised, tensions within the *Annales* way of doing medical history. Conceived along the lines of a Braudelian *enquête* into material life, Peter's analysis shifted to the epistemological concerns associated with Foucault's work on medicine as discourse and as power. Peter provided a sort of archival gloss or subtext to Foucault's conclusions from published material on the transformation of Paris medicine and psychiatry and the constitution of medical power before and during the time of the Revolution. The 'Malades et maladies' article of 1967 confronted the *Annales* with what might be called the uncertainty problem in medical historiography: how could one rely on medical history as a technique when that technique was in fact a discipline with an internal problematic evident in its own complex evolving history?

No consensus on how to deal with this problem has emerged, at least not within the *Annales*. The disease *enquête* under the auspices of the VIe section was confided to Jean-Paul Aron, Peter, and Jean-Pierre Goubert and expanded to an even more ambitious investigation into medicine and medical practitioners in France over the past two centuries. But the project collapsed in the mid 1970s, apparently due to lack of funds. It seems likely that unresolved tensions about how medical history should be done, tensions visible in the Peter article and which I have characterised as Braudelian versus Foucaultian, may have had something to do with the untimely demise of the disease *enquête*. In any case, there were no further publications under its direct auspices. Peter's full-length study of the Société Royale did not (and has not yet) appeared and his subsequent publications were not in the *Annales*.[32]

The 1970s were nonetheless a rich decade for medical historiography in the *Annales*. Gone was the earlier monolithic devotion to biology, demography and epidemiology, although these approaches remained well represented (11 of 20 articles). Indeed they were strengthened by the increasing participation of specialists from the bio-medical sciences and physical anthropology. A general movement toward anthropology and ethnology by the *Annales* also found expression in several articles on medical ethnology.[33] Six contributions appeared on the history of psychiatry, in part evidence of Foucault's impact, and also that of psycho-history, to which the *Annales* devoted a special section in March-April 1973.[34] In addition there were articles on the history of ideas about brain psychology (1970), medical epistemology (1975), women and medicine (1976) and religious healing (1976). All of this showed the openness of the *Annales* to new themes in historiography without necessarily reflecting any broader commitment. The *Annales* of the 1970s had become eclectic.

In 1977, a special number devoted to history of medicine included ten articles grouped into three divisions: 'doctors in society,' 'doctors and [other] healers' and 'medical discourse and practice'. As these headings suggested, the special number dealt with territory familiar to medical historians. Such topics had seldom found space in the journal before and, it might be added, rarely since. In a sense, the special number of the *Annales* represented official if belated recognition of the social history of medicine, a field cultivated in France for at least a decade, but not nearly as actively as in Great Britain and North America. I have discussed elsewhere the contents of the September-October 1977 *Annales*.[35] Here, I shall limit myself to what it seemed to represent in the context of the *Annales*' perception of medical history.

Jacques Revel, as editorial spokesman for the *Annales*, wrote a preface to the special number. Somewhat ambiguously, Revel welcomed the history of medicine and disease as a discipline which, although neither new nor interdisciplinary and indeed somewhat narrow, nevertheless 'did not strike us as too bad a terrain' for an *enquête* and for historical reflection. Previously the closed fiefdom of 'erudite or curious medical doctors', it had become an enterprise worthy of broader historical investigation.[36]

Indeed, none of the contributors to the special number were medical doctors, although several, like Jacques Léonard and Jean-Pierre Goubert, had published extensively enough in the field to deserve the status of specialists in this particular area of social history. Others like Jacques Gélis and Mireille Laget had drawn upon doctorats d'état and monographs in preparation. Revel attributed the upsurge of interest in medical history to two factors I have already noted, the oeuvre of Foucault and the archival treasure trove of the Société Royale de Médecine. Thirdly, Revel invoked a raised cultural sensitivity (in which Foucault had played a role despite his personal absence from Paris during the crisis of 1968) to 'institutions of social control', among which medicine figured prominently. Several of the articles in the *Annales* number drew heavily upon the Société Royale source; virtually all were situated against the Foucaultian chronology and context of a late-18th-century medical epistemological 'rupture'. Many showed an awareness of *pouvoir médical* but only Farge on artisans' diseases and, in a more muted way, Léonard on nurses, Goubert on charlatans, and Gélis on midwives sounded a note critical of medicalisation.

The special number of 1977 marked a culmination of *Annales* interest in the history of medicine, a recognition that subjects previously deemed parochial and left to physician-historians, problems of medical professional organisation, status, values and institutions needed to be woven into the ambitious project that Revel called 'the constitution of a physical anthropology of the past'. It is still too early to say whether the *Annales* of the 1980s will be open to the social and intellectual history of medicine. Most of the work published since 1977, it should be noted (ten articles), fits rather the older Braudelian tendency to equate medicine with the bio-demographic side of history.

Figure 1.2 summarises the general pattern of the contents of *Annales* medical history. Thirty-eight articles published since 1947 (leaving aside for the moment the two special numbers) may be broken down into the following categories: demography-epidemiology (14 articles), biology-physical anthropology (7), psychiatry (6), ethnology (6), and history of science and ideas (5). Adding in the special number of 1969 raises the total on demography-epidemiology to 18, biology-physical anthropology to 9 and ethnology to 6; the contributions to the special number of 1977, as noted, did not fit into these categories, but were devoted to the history of the profession, institutions, practice and patients.

There are, of course, articles that might be assigned to more than one category. Peter's article, discussed above, although primarily epidemiological (and counted as such) also dealt with history of ideas and ethnology; conversely I judged Esoavelomandroso's recent article on resistance to plague measures in colonial Madagascar to be ethnological despite much epidemiological

Figure 1.2: Annales: *Content by subcategory of medical history. Hatched area represents Nov.-Dec. 1969*

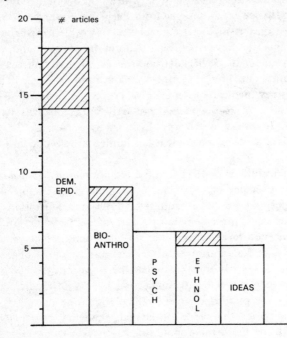

content. Several other articles on epidemics gave varying degrees of attention to ethnology or *mentalité*.[37]

Despite these and other problems of classification, the predominant theme of medical historiography in the *Annales* appears clearly to be the history of material life: since 1960 27 articles where as against seven on ethnology. Articles on the history of science and ideas have not only been rare but their authors have been for the most part marginal to the *Annales* nerve centre in the Ecole Pratique des Hautes Etudes en Sciences Sociales and have had little in common with the mainstream of *Annales* historiography.[38]

This is particularly striking when one looks at the six articles on psychiatry, all published between 1970 and 1975. Of these, only two, I think, would be recognised as owing any debt to an *Annales* approach to history. They are Peter Burke's introductory sketch to a social history of dreams and, to a lesser extent, Michel de Certeau's epistemological analysis of Freud's discussion of a 17th-century case of demonic possession as neurosis. Both articles, despite the psychoanalytic choice of subject matter, employ methods of comparative ethnology and the study of mentalité in ways seen elsewhere in the *Annales*, and both authors have been associated with other *Annales* projects. The situation is quite different with the remaining four articles on psychiatry. Gérard Bleandonu and Guy Le Gaufey, writing on the birth of mental asylums in 19th-century Auxerre and Paris (1975), explicitly invoke Foucault's book on madness as their point of departure. They go on to demonstrate how short-term changes in 'economic and social conjuncture' and elite individual historical actors, such as Baron Haussmann, determined the type of asylums constructed. Like Bleandonu and Le Gaufey, Georges Lanteri-Laura, then a psychiatrist at Strasbourg University, in his study on chronic diseases in 19th-century French psychiatry (1972), drew upon history of ideas and socio-economic history. Finally, Aurigemma's article on Jung and Carl Schorske's on Freud appear not to have been originally contributed to the *Annales* but rather republished by that journal in French translation. In any case, both essays concentrated on cultural and intellectual biography.

By now it should be clear that the *Annales*, as far as medical history is concerned, has remained remarkably faithful to the Braudelian prescription of building upon material structures. Indeed, there has been a definite tendency to go beyond what Braudel practised in medical history (demographic and epidemiological)[39] to what he preached (biological and pathological). Making their presence felt in the pages of the *Annales* were historians of the bio-medical sciences like Dr Mirko Grmek of the IV[e] section of the EPHE, contributor of three articles between 1963 and 1975 and, more recently, specialists in haematology and population biology, notably Jean Bernard and Jacques Ruffier, co-authors of two articles (1976, 1979).

In contrast to Braudel's enduring influence, the legacy of the founders, Marc Bloch and Lucien Febvre, is much less discernible. Only two articles on miracle healing followed Bloch's precedent, and Febvre's zeal for the history of high culture, including medical and scientific ideas, was in effect rejected by *Annales* medical historiography.

In addition to a content heavily skewed toward material life, the context of the medical history articles has also been archetypically Braudelian. Nine of the 38 articles sweep across long periods of time or are difficult to situate in any conventional chronological niche. Of the remainder, seven deal with the ancient/mediaeval/early modern periods; nine with 'modern' in the French sense, i.e. the 17th and 18th centuries; nine with the 19th century; and four with the 20th century.[40] If one leaves aside two articles published in 1947 and 1952 and the work on history of ideas and psychiatry already seen to be outside the mainstream, the 19th-century component is reduced to just two articles — both on the cholera epidemics.[41]

The *Annales* virtual exclusion of 'modern' history in the Anglo-American sense of the word is confirmed in the two special numbers: that of 1969 contains one *longue durée* article, four ancient/mediaeval/early modern, one 18th century, and one 18th–19th century; that of 1977, its misleading title reference to the 18th and 19th centuries notwithstanding, devotes eight of ten articles to the Old Regime; one other deals with the consulate and empire and only one article — by Jacques Léonard on nursing sisters — ventures into the post-Napoleonic 19th century.

Jacques Léonard is clearly one of the leading current exponents of the social and cultural history of medicine in 19th-century France. His links with the *Annales* tradition are somewhat ambiguous but he shares a preference for a quantitative empirical approach to economic and social history and he has made frequent contributions as a reviewer to the *Annales*.[42] Yet the complete absence of references to the *Annales* in the bibliographical essay on secondary sources in Léonard's recent study of 19th-century French medicine (*La médecine entre les savoirs et les pouvoirs* (1981)) serves further to confirm that the journal has had little to offer in this respect. Given Léonard's own background as an historian, it is somewhat surprising to find that nearly half of his 29 citations are to books by medical doctors and ten to works written before 1960. Whoever has dealt with medicine in post-revolutionary France, clearly it has not been the *Annales*.

Why have the *Annales* shunned 19th-century medicine and with it so much of importance for understanding modern culture? Why do the names and scientific upheavals associated with Louis Pasteur, Claude Bernard, and Jean-Martin Charcot, to take only the three best-known French medical symbols of the century, not appear? In principle, the answers are self-evident. Such subjects are the stuff of traditional events history, the rapid history of short-term change preoccupied with personalities, politics, and conscious ideas. Much of the material reviewed in the preceding pages constitutes the *Annales* response and alternative to that kind of history.

It is time, however, to call in question the *Annales* neglect of almost two centuries of recent medical history as well as history in general.[43] For this, of course, we must return to the commanding figure of Fernand Braudel. In his classic formulation of the *longue durée* in 1958, Braudel, in effect, ruled that any historian of the contemporary period who did not extend his story back until at least the first half of the preceding century would fail to meet the criterion of the *longue durée*; i.e. to look at time periods at least one century in duration. By implication, then, an historian of the Third Republic could at best aspire to medium-term or conjunctural history, if not the analysis of short-term change best left to 'chroniclers and journalists'.[44] Elsewhere, Braudel castigated the demographic historian, Louis Chevalier, for, among other things, not looking at a long enough period in his study of the Parisian poor during the first half of the 19th century.[45]

Braudel, nevertheless, in the spirit of Febvre, maintained a keen interest in the relation between present and past, and he encouraged *Annales* publications in 'history of the present', a rubric often devoted to the developing or third world. As far as Western civilisation was concerned, Braudel suggested that the present began around 1750, presumably an allusion to the demographic and industrial revolutions.[46] If this reading of Braudel is accurate (allowing for schematic simplification), *longue durée* historiography and with it a full structural approach to history reaches a dead end sometime before the 19th century. Braudel's temporal definitions inevitably lead to this conclusion.

It appears likely that the very *concept* of *longue durée*, as well as its temporal applicability, meets an impasse with the industrial era. Braudel's formulation of the concept reflected his experience as an historian of the early modern period. His view of 'societies for whom a day, a year doesn't mean much, for whom, at times, an entire century is only of an instant's duration' becomes almost meaningless for industrial and subsequent societies.[47] The relation of man with the earth, for Braudel a rapport 'out of the reach and the bite of time', has in fact been subjected to the continual transformation by new technologies. Since the end of the 18th century, the environment and the biological nature of man have escaped millenial steady-state equilibria.[48] Furthermore, as Henk L. Wesseling has remarked, modern politics became mass politics and, therefore, a fundamental structure of modern social history in a way that older political history was not.[49]

The *Annales* preoccupation with pre-industrial societies, thus, while it may not be an irrevocable philosophical commitment, did arise out of research interests and imperatives of its founders, Febvre, Bloch, and Braudel, the colleagues and students they recruited to their enterprise, and the great majority of the historians, past and present, they singled out for praise. Like begets like. Even so, it is surprising that even now, long after Braudel's withdrawal from active direction of the journal, and when the *longue durée* has ceased to be dogma, that the *Annales* remains reluctant in practice if not in principle to cross the traditional threshold of the French Revolution and enter the 19th century. On the other hand, there is enthusiasm for 'history of the present' (with which 20th- and sometimes even 19th-century history are conflated) even if it is typically left for superior journalists and practitioners of the other human sciences.[50]

I see no reason why historians of the 19th century need resign themselves to the constraints of events history. The social science approaches to history pioneered by the *Annales* and possibly even a modified form of *longue durée* structural analysis can find fruitful application to 19th-century history generally and to medical history in particular. Indeed, to return to medical history, the process has already begun with Annalistes and fellow-traveller historians like Léonard, Alain Corbin, Olivier Faure, Jean-Pierre Goubert, and others.[51]

The *bilan* of the *Annales*, in medical history, this paper has argued, has been moulded by epistemological assumptions that restricted the majority of articles published on the subject within the confines of material history. What then of its *perspectives*? Prediction is, of course, much more hazardous than retrospective analysis. The history of the *Annales* enterprise itself illustrates this precept. Since this paper was read, important changes in the direction of *Annales* have proceeded apace. Fernand Braudel's death in 1985 may prove to be more than a symbol of the end of era in the scientistic orientation of a review he did so much to raise to pre-eminence. It is possible that the accelerating attention to anthropologically informed historiography in recent years will encourage looking at the body, disease and medicine in ways that 'harder', more positivistic social sciences such as demography, economics and sociology did not readily permit. A perceptible resurgence of narrative and even broadly conceived political and cultural history within the *Annales* might also promote the cultural history of medicine.

The *Annales*, of course, is not required to be all things to all people and certainly not to all historians of medicine. If it has failed to address conceptual and intellectual problems customarily dealt with by historians of medicine and science, and has been somewhat retrograde with regard to the new social history of medicine, that is its privilege and, doubtless, its choice. As Fernand Braudel and others have remarked, the *Annales*, since about the mid-1960s, has had to live with a heavy burden it did not bear during the earlier years, that of being so successful that it became the orthodox historical establishment, the object of great praise, but, then, also inevitably the target of criticism.

Notes

1. See J.H. Hexter, 'Fernand Braudel and the *Monde* Braudellien . . .' *Journal of Modern History, 44* (1972), 480–539.
2. British and North American historians of French medicine who come to mind as more or less influenced by the *Annales* are: William Coleman, Toby Gelfand, Caroline Hannaway, Colin Jones, Harvey Mitchell, Terence D. Murphy, Matthew Ramsey and George Sussman.
3. Lucien Febvre, *La terre et l'évolution humaine* (Paris, 1970 1st edn. 1922), 390.
4. Fernand Braudel, 'En guise de conclusion', *Review, 1* (1978), 247.
5. Jacques Revel, 'Histoire et sciences sociales: Les Paradigmes des Annales', *Annales: E.S.C., 34* (1979), 1360–76, esp. p. 1361.
6. E.H. Ackerknecht, 'A plea for a "Behaviorist" Approach in writing the History of Medicine', *Journal of the History of Medicine, 22* (1967), 211–14.
7. F. Lebrun, *Les hommes et la mort en Anjou aux XVIIe et XVIIIe siècles. Essai de démographie et de psychologie historiques* (Paris-La Haye, 1971); J.-P. Goubert, *Malades et médecins en Bretagne 1770–1790* (Paris, 1974); J. Léonard, *Les médecins de l'oeust au XIXe siècle,* 3 vols. (Lille, 1976); J.-N. Biraben, *Les hommes et la peste en France et dans les pays européens et méditerranéans* (Paris, 1975); F. Loux, *Le jeune enfant et son corps dans la médecine traditionnelle* (Paris, 1978); V.-P. Comiti, *La géographie médicale de la Corse à la fin du XVIIIe siècle* (Geneve, 1980); M. Laget, *Naissance, L'accouchement avant l'âge de la Clinique* (Paris, 1982); M.-C. Pouchelle, *Corps et chirurgie à l'apogée du moyen âge* (Paris, 1983); Jacques Gélis, *L'arbre et le fruit: la naissance dans l'occident moderne (XVIe–XIXe siècle)* (Paris, 1984).
8. 'A nos lecteurs', *Annales d'histoire économique et sociale, 1* (1929), 1–2.
9. Febvre, 'Contre l'esprit de spécialité, Une lettre de 1933', in Lucien Febvre, *Combats pour l'histoire* (Paris, 1953), 104–6.
10. P. Goubert, *Beauvais et le Beauvaisis de 1600 à 1730* (Paris, 1960), 69–75; G. Frêche, *Toulouse et la région midi-Pyrénées au siècle des lumières (vers 1670–1789)* (Paris, 1974), 95–120; J.-C. Perrot, *Génèse d'une ville moderne. Caen au XVIIIe siècle* (Paris, 1975), vol. 2, 882–943. Although his thèse d'état, *Les Paysans de Languedoc,* 2 vols. (Paris, 1966) scarcely mentioned disease or medicine, Le Roy Ladurie emerged in the mid- and late 1960s as one of the most powerful advocates within the *Annales* school of a

bio-medical approach to history. See various articles collected in his *Le Territoire de l'Historien* (Paris, 1973), esp. pp. 59–61, 80–6, 301–415, and 'Un concept: l'unification microbienne du monde (XIVe–XVIIe siècles)', *Revue Suisse de l'Histoire, 23* (1973), 627–96.

11. Measured in terms of page volume (leaving aside the special numbers), the *Annales* medical history articles constituted the following percentages of total page volume: 1950s, 0.5 per cent; 1960s, 1.3 per cent; 1970s, 2.6 per cent; 1980s (to July-August 1984), 2.3 per cent.

12. Febvre, in *Combats pour l'histoire*, pp. 245, 314–36.

13. Significantly, no mention of Sarton nor Sigerist turns up in the index of the *Annales: E.S.C.* for the period 1929–1951.

14. Febvre, in *Combats pour l'histoire,* pp. 334–6. The book under review was Henri Daudin, *Etudes d'histoire des sciences naturelles,* 3 vols. (Paris, 1926).

15. For example, Febvre reviewed three books by medical doctors: R. Dumesnil, *Histoire illustrée de la médecine* (in *Annales d'Histoire Economique et Sociale, 8* (1936), 181); P. Delaunay, *La vie médicale aux XVIe, XVIIe et XVIIIe siècles* (in ibid. *8* (1936), 180–1); and R. Mercier, *Le monde médical de Tourraine sous la Révolution* (ibid., *11* (1939), 82). In the review of Delaunay (1936), Febvre candidly expressed his view that satisfactory medical historiography of the future would require collaboration between social historians, medical doctors, and philosophers: 'Tant que nous n'aurons pas des études fortement bassés sur une telle collaboration (je dis collaboration et non juxtaposition), nous aurons des histoires sur la médecine, plus ou moins sérieuses, plus on moins pénétrantes et documentées; nous n'aurons pas d'histoires de la médecine'.

Insight into the receptivity of the *Annales* to medical history might be gained by an analysis of their book reviews of work in the discipline over the years. A preliminary survey by Lorraine O'Donnell, my research assistant at the University of Ottawa, suggests a very restrained interest indeed: during the period 1949–1968, fewer than ten books in medical history were selected for review; the dismissive titles of several reviews such as 'une histoire anecdotique' (*9* (1954), 279) or 'petite histoire' (*11* (1956), 424) provide glimpses into editorial attitudes toward the works in question, if not the field in general. Between 1969 and 1985 the number of reviews increased to about 30 (reflecting the special interests of historians like Jacques Léonard and Jean-Pierre Goubert who wrote nearly one-third of these reviews) but the total, of course, represents but a minute fraction of books published in the field. At a conference of medical historians in 1986, for example, 250 'recent' books were exhibited. *AAHM Newsletter American Association for the History of Medicine*, no. 21 (Summer, 1986).

16. Callot failed to mention the important monograph on the problem published just two years earlier by E.H. Ackerknecht, *Malaria in the Upper Mississippi Valley* (Baltimore, 1945) in which a similar interpretation was sustained.

17. *Annales: E.S.C., 16* (1961), 423–4.

18. Ibid., pp. 545–6.

19. *Annales E.S.C., 24* (Nov.-Dec., 1969), preface.

20. For a muted protest against the view of mentalité as merely something added on to the upper layers of the total history project, see

Robert Mandrou, 'Histoire sociale et histoire des mentalités', *La Nouvelle Critique* (Jan. 1972), 41–4, esp. p. 44. An explicit criticism of Braudel for neglecting the realm of 'ideas, religion, mental attitudes, cognitive structures' is made by Keith Thomas, *The New York Review of Books* (December 13, 1973), 4.

21. For a perceptive essay in this sense, see Allan Megill, 'Foucault, structuralism, and the ends of history', *Journal of Modern History, 51* (1979), 451–503.

22. See, for example, 'Foucault et les historiens, entretien avec Jacques Revel', *Magazine littéraire* (June 1975), 10–13; Roger Chartier, 'Les chemins de l'histoire', *Le Nouvel Observateur* (June 29, 1984), 56, both written largely from the perspective of what Foucault has done to and for historiography. For medical historiography, see remarks by J.-P. Goubert in L. G. Stevenson (ed.), *A Celebration of Medical History* (Baltimore, 1982), 157–8 and Caroline Hannaway, ibid., pp. 177–8.

23. Farge, 'Face à l'histoire', *Magazine littéraire* (May 1984), 40–2.

24. *Review* 1 (1978), 256; Foucault's only contribution to the *Annales* was, significantly, a critique of a study in literary biography, not an historical piece in the usual sense: 'Le Mallarmé de J.-P. Richard', *Annales: E.S.C., 19* (1964), 996–1004. In 1968, Braudel referred to Foucault as one of 'the structuralists of the new literary criticism'. *International Encyclopedia of the Social Sciences, 5,* 349. Braudel promised 'a long critical article on the oeuvre of Michel Foucault' to *Le Nouvel Observateur.* See *Le Nouvel Observateur* (June 29, 1984), 55, but it evidently was never published.

25. *Annales: E.S.C., 17* (1962), 761–71. In a postscript, Braudel added his own high praise of Foucault's achievement, ibid., pp. 771–2.

26. Peter, 'Malades et maladies à la fin du XVIIIe siècle', *Annales: E.S.C., 22* (1967), 711–51. Page references to this article will be to its reprinted version in *Médecins, Climat et Epidémies,* pp. 135–70 and to its English translation 'Disease and the sick at the end of the eighteenth century', in R. Forster and O. Ranum (eds), *Biology of Man in History. Selections from the Annales,* trans. by E. Forster and P. M. Ranum (Baltimore, 1975), 81–124. Peter's contrast between 'geology' and 'archaeology' is in *Médecins, Climat,* p. 139.

27. Foucault's *L'Archéologie du Savoir* would appear in 1969. Peter participated in Foucault's seminar at the Collège de France and worked on the *équipe* responsible for the publication of *Moi, Pierre Rivière ayant égorgé ma mère, ma soeur et mon frère . . . un cas de parricide au XIXe siècle.* Collection Archives (Paris, 1973).

28. Peter, 'Disease and the sick', in Forster and Ranum (eds.), *Biology of Man,* p. 94.

29. Peter, 'Maladies et malades', in *Médecins, Climat,* p. 150.

30. Peter, 'Disease and the sick', in Forster and Ranum (eds.), *Biology of Man,* p. 107.

31. Ibid., p. 117.

32. Peter's approach may indeed have provoked the discontent of Braudel to the point where the young historian was virtually 'exiled' from the *Annales.* His next publication on the Société Royale de Médecine, 'Les mots et les aspects de la maladie' appeared in the more traditionalist and

less prestigious *Revue historique, 499* (1971), 13–38. (Personal intervention by Jean-Pierre Goubert at Cambridge Conference, March 1985.)

For the aspirations of the disease enquête, see its programme in J.-P. Aron, J.-P. Goubert and J.-P. Peter, 'La médecine et les médecins en France depuis deux siècles, Nouvelles Enquête', *Démographie historique*, no. 11 (1974), 15–21. The medical sections of the monograph, *Médecins, Climat et Epidémies* (Paris, 1972) simply reprinted previously published articles. Peter mentioned the prospect of a second volume (p. 135) but it never appeared. In addition Le Roy Ladurie, who invoked the full support of Braudel for the enquête, expected a forthcoming book by Peter (*Médecins, Climat*, pp. 5–6.). Peter's subsequent publications increasingly emphasised ethnological and epistemological perspectives rather than epidemiology. See e.g. 'Le corps du délit', *Nouvelle revue de psychoanalyse, 3* (1971), 71–108 and 'Entre femmes et médecins', *Ethnologie française, 6* (1976), 341–8. Perhaps his clearest statement of dissatisfaction with the way in which history of disease had been written as the 'natural history of disease' came in an article co-authored with Jacques Revel, 'Le corps: l'homme malade et son histoire', in J. Legoff and P. Nora (eds.), *Faire de l'histoire*, vol. 3 (1974), 169–91.

33. See André Burguière, 'The New Annales: A redefinition of the late 1960s', *Review, 1* (1978), 195–205.

34. 'Histoire et psychoanalyse', *Annales: E.S.C., 28* (1973), 309–67.

35. T. Gelfand, 'The Annales and the History of Medicine', *Bulletin of the History of Medicine, 55* (1981), 589–93.

36. Revel, *Annales: E.S.C., 32* (1977), 849–50.

37. See e.g. R. Baehrel, 'La Haine de classe en temps d'epidémie', *Annales: E.S.C., 7* (1952), 351–60; Catherine Rollet and Agnès Souriac, 'Epidémies et mentalités: le cholera de 1832 en Seine et Oise', ibid., *29* (1974), 935–65.

38. See e.g. François Le Plassotte, 'Quelques étapes de la physiologie du cerveau du XVIIe au début du XIXe siècle', ibid., *25* (1970), 599–613; Claire Soloman-Bayet, 'L'Institution de la science: un exemple au XVIIIe siècle', ibid., *30* (1975), 1028–44. La Plassotte was in the department of psychology at the University of Clermont and Solomon-Bayet at the Institute of history of sciences at the CNRS.

39. Braudel, *The Mediterranean and the Mediterranean World in the Age of Phillip II*, trans. Sian Reynolds, 2 vols. (London, 1972), 258–9, 332–4; *Civilisation matérielle et capitalisme*, vol. 1, pp. 51–68.

40. A glance at Anglo-American social history of medicine shows quite different chronological foci of interest with the bulk of work dealing with developments after 1800. See e.g. *Bulletins of the Society for the Social History of Medicine* (United Kingdom) 1969–1985, *passim*. For a systematic comparison between *Annales* and other general historical journals on periodisation, see H.L. Wesseling, 'The *Annales* school and the writing of contemporary history', *Review, 1* (1978), 185–94.

41. Rollet and Souriac, 'Epidémies et mentalités: le cholera de 1832 en Seine et Oise'; Patrice Bourdelais and Jean-Yves Raulot, 'Le marche du cholera en France, 1832 et 1854', *Annales: E.S.C., 33* (1978), 125–42. Both articles drew upon the pioneering study by Louis Chevalier, 'Paris' in L. Chevalier (ed.), *Le Cholera: la premier epidémie du XIXe siècle* (Paris,

1958), 3–45. Chevalier's brilliant precedent none the less had curiously little direct impact upon medical historiography in the *Annales*. Perhaps Braudel's severe critique of Chevalier's *Classes laborieuses et classes dangereuses à Paris dans la première moitié du XIXe siècle* (Paris, 1958), in which the cholera material also appeared, was responsible. Braudel found Chevalier guilty on three main counts: demographic 'imperialism', excessive reliance on literary sources, and limiting his discussion to the 19th century. See Braudel, *Ecrits sur l'histoire* (Paris, 1969), 220–35.

42. See Matthew Ramsey, 'Review essay: history of a profession, *Annales* style: the work of Jacques Léonard', *Journal of Social History, 17* (1984), 319–38. For Léonard's objections to Foucault's approach to history, see his essay 'L'historien et le philosophe' in M. Perrot (ed.), *L'Impossible Prison* (Paris, 1980), 9–28.

43. See H.L. Wesseling, 'The *Annales* School and the writing of contemporary history', *Review, 1* (1978), 185–94.

44. Braudel, 'Histoire et sciences sociales. La *longue durée* (1958)' in *Ecrits sur l'histoire* (Paris, 1969), 41–83, esp. p. 46.

45. Ibid., p. 233. Braudel wrote the review of Chevalier's book in 1960.

46. Ibid., p. 309 ('L'Histoire des civilisations: le passé explique le présent', 1959).

47. Ibid., p. 24 ('Préface, la Méditerranée et le monde Méditerranéen à l'epoque de Philippe II', 1949).

48. Braudel acknowledges this chronological limit to the *longue-durée* in an example taken from the history of disease. See *Civilisation matérielle*, vol. 1, 67–8.

49. Wesseling, pp. 192–4.

50. See Pierre Nora, 'Présent' in J. Legoff, R. Chartier and J. Revel (eds.), *La Nouvelle Histoire* (Paris, 1978), 467–72.

51. Léonard, in Perrot (ed.), *L'Impossible Prison*; Corbin, *Les filles de noce, Misère sexuelle et prostitution aux 19e et 20e siècles* (Paris, 1978); Corbin, *Le miasme et la jonquille. L'odorat et l'imaginaire social XVIIIe–XIXe siècles* (Paris, 1982); Faure, *Génèse de l'hôpital moderne: les hôpitaux civils de Lyon de 1802* (Lyon, 1981). J.-P. Goubert 'La conquête de l'eau. Analyse historique du rapport à l'eau dans le France contemporaine' (thèse d'état soutenue 3 fév. 1984). In addition Marc Ferro and Jean-Paul Aron have made a film on the history of medicine that deals with modern transformations of old problems and with problems created by new technologies.

2

Twenty Years On: Problems of Historical Methodology in the History of Health*

J.-P. Goubert

Exactly twenty-two years ago, while still a young student, I was tackling questions pertaining to the history of health.[1] At that time, I took as my model my great predecessors: my own father, who was one of the two founders of historical demography in France; but also Philippe Ariès, François Lebrun and Michel Vovelle, who were beginning to study, with talent and perspicacity, the history of death in Western societies.

Trained in social history (and not in the history of mentalities or that of science), I did not have a very 'philosophical' mind. The history of ideas, practised by certain North American and German colleagues, seemed old hat to me then, almost a relic of the Dark Ages. I strongly believed — as I no doubt needed to — in a renewal of the history of health by social history, the methods of which seemed surer and better tested. Alienated from the history of ideas and from a conceptualisation that, to me, was equivalent to abstraction, I was equally alienated from Parisian intellectual fashions, personified by the success of a Michel Foucault with 'his' history of madness and 'his' birth of the clinic. These assignations, like the ill-treatment to which he subjected history, alienated me then from his methodological practices and from the spirit that marked them. I believed — and I still believe — in the existence of clear and comprehensible thought; I excluded obscurantism and 'superstition', whereas today I seize upon them. As a worthy heir of the French ideology issuing from the Third Republic, I reviled a certain number of values considered as conservative, indeed as reactionary. I was not only indifferent, but above all hostile to the intellectual contribution made by Freudian and post-

* Translated by George St Andrews

Freudian psychoanalysis. It seemed impossible to me that discoveries of this type could be applied to former times, or still more,
to social groups.

At this period of my life I practised, without being too aware
of it, a positive or even positivist history, fortunately counter-
balanced by a solid criticism of the sources (in the old way, which
had some good in it) and by a sometimes superficial scepticism.
I was imbued with a number of *a priori* concepts and ready-made
ideas. Thus, I took up the contempt of the medical world of my
time for charlatans, without conceiving that the veil of contempt
hid from me the treasures of a popular culture that, although it
had different criteria and modes of expression, was in the end just
as 'logical'. I had been brought up in the midst of the 'historical
seraglio', almost without a glance to spare for certain other social
sciences, particularly anthropology. On the other hand, I knew
quite a lot about historical 'periods', and even about geography
(mostly, human). Sociology was not wholly unknown to me and
I was familiar with historical demography. Finally, I had a vivid
and real sympathy for those who suffer, whatever their social
milieu.

I was confident of the certitudes of my youth and was also
imbued with certain prejudices stemming from my education and
my temperament. Jean Meyer then managed to find the topic for
a Diplôme d'Etudes Supérieures that suited me: mortality in
Brittany at the end of the eighteenth century.[2] It enabled me to
plunge into the very rich administrative archives of Brittany at the
end of the *Ancien Régime*. This also gave me the chance to practise
historical demography with respect to the 'crises of mortality' and,
still more, to understand to what extent death (the phenomenon,
not its image) is the child and the product of its time, and to what
extent the expiring *Ancien Régime* was incapable of resolving the
crucial problems of the age, including that of physiological and
social misery.

To reconstitute a period, to retell a 'bit' of history, to grasp life
in suspension, to diagnose — if possible — the maladies of yesterday in today's terms — such questions absorbed my time and my
reflections. Neither actor in, nor spectator of the story being told,
I used to reconstruct the 'drama' from signs and testimonies,
without always noticing then that the montage thus effected often
resulted from my personal mode of intellectual functioning.

In any case, one thing that I still today regard as essential is the
patient work of reconstruction in the domain of public health,

starting from a solid socio-demographic base. In this way one has some chance of describing the ways of life of a whole population or else of certain social groups. If one is unaware that the majority of the Breton population were rural, that they lived poorly, if not often in destitution, that they could not afford the luxury of calling a doctor or of paying for cinchona (quinine), one can have little conception of the very real difficulties faced there by scientific medicine, coming from the well-to-do world of the town and a written, 'enlightened' culture, rejecting fatalism the better to affirm the possibilities of knowledge and its grasp on 'reality'.

I hope I will be forgiven this rather long and very egocentric introduction. Arriving at a turning-point in his life, the historian, like so many others, feels the need to give it meaning. He becomes his own observer. To separate the history in the writing from the historian 'in the making' has always seemed an aberration to me, one of those 'sectors' of the unsaid and the clandestine, as Guy Thuillier likes to call them.[3] To render this a rather more academic account, I will distinguish three types of methodological problems: (1) The general problem of the particular prejudices of the historian; (2) the problem of the sources used, of their origins, and their 'silences' and (3) the problems specific to a historical study of public health.

The historian's prejudices

Questions of place and time, quite obviously, play a paramount part. Brittany cannot truly be studied without taking into consideration, with the help of some great geographers like Maurice Le Lannou and Vidal de la Blache,[4] its peninsular position, the Armorican massif, the Breton moorlands and the interior basins, the coast that is mostly rocky and fringed with deep estuaries. Similarly, recourse to the ethnographers of yesterday and today proves to be essential for anyone who wants to understand the cultural atmosphere or 'the attitudes of the Bretons in the face of death'.[5] The Celtic imagination, the fear of the Ankou, and the rituals of the exorcism cannot be separated from an analysis attentive to attitudes to death and illness.

The question of period also plays an essential role. In so far as one is dealing with the pre-revolutionary period (1770–1789), several major risks exist that one must strive to avoid.[6] One consists in regarding the Revolution as the necessary 'terminus ad quem' of a long period, that of the *Ancien Régime*. Another, perhaps still more serious, stems from giving legitimacy to one of the periods of the French Revolution to the detriment of the others: the *Ancien Régime* is held up against the Revolution (or the other way round), the principles of '89' against the first Republic (and vice versa), to give but two examples.

In the second place, other prejudices, while indeed less evident to certain people, are but the more serious in their effects. This time, there is a double risk. When it comes to expressing oneself on a subject that concerns medicine, public health and medical care, particularly in France, there is a risk of falling into two exactly parallel excesses: that of praise, which sometimes verges on the hagiography of the medical world, and that of hyper-criticism, which mixes up civilised society (société policée) and police state (société policière) and which sometimes sees the origins of totalitarianism in the Enlightenment.

With regard to the medical world, to the ladies of charity, the clergy and the throng of therapists (learned as well as popular) let us not forget that, whatever their respective merits, they expected a 'return', a recompense, a reciprocity: be it here below, in the form of gratitude, of legitimation, of honoraria, or in the other world, with an open door to Heaven.

Incontestably, the greatest error into which the historian can fall consists in judging the values of yesterday or the day before yesterday with the yardstick of the values of our time. We can do better than this: we must seize, understand, unravel the threads of the inextricable, and then clarify, explain, narrate, popularise (in the good sense of the term). Our task is to bring to light the 'original characteristics' of a vast province, to describe its levels of health, recount its 'wisdoms of the body', either common or particular to a part of the social body.

A historical sociology and anthropology of difference are thus necessary. It is not enough to make a quantitative estimate of the alimentary ration, to stress the imbalance of the diet, to denounce the lack of hygiene in having hospital beds occupied by several patients, and to stigmatise the impotence of pre-scientific medicine. We must also — and therein lies our task as historians — come to grips with a society of the past as something other than just the negation or the absence of ours. Hence, we must observe which social and cultural mechanisms have given rise to the situations analysed: for example, we must grasp that the idea of contagion was not known, not only among the lower classes but also among many élites, and that moreover, sleeping several to a bed at the time of epidemics was a custom that allowed bodies to keep warm (in the absence of central heating!), not to mention the fact that the finances of hospitals were often in a parlous state at this period.

To avoid repeating the discourse of the hygienists without submitting it to historical criticism; to look for the foundations of our epidemic and emotional reactions; to grasp the origins and the causes of socio-cultural change; not to stay buried in the archives but to establish a balance-sheet of what they tell us and what they hide from us, particularly in such delicate areas as those of the relations between health, illness and money[7] — such are, to my mind, the principles, simple to state but more difficult to put into practice, that can guide the informed researcher in the field of the history of health. To be attentive to the 'silences of history', according to Jacques le Goff's formula, necessitates an attention and a concentration that form part of the definition of true 'craftmanship'. Thus, pinpointing the different usages of the term superstition from the pen of 'enlightened' doctors and administrators clearly shows that what is involved here is a value-judgement about the nature of knowledge and, in particular, that of practical medicine: the quack is contemptible because he exploits the superstitions of his clients. He is outside the dominant culture and, for that reason, exposes it to ridicule.[8] Consequently, moral condemnation of the quack has prevented a number of doctors, past and present, and also certain historians, from seeing that 'quackery' and 'superstitions' with regard to the body obey a system of values and representations that has its own authenticity. To limit oneself to condemning the bone-setter for practising medicine illegally is the concern of the law and its applications, not the historian's work. The same goes for the old practice of women giving mutual help when one of them gave birth. We have in this a social and cultural phenomenon of ancient date that an anthropological approach helps to throw light on. The birth of a man's child is women's business. The reciprocity of services tightens the bonds of the female part of the village community. It also highlights the work of 'fructification' carried out in the bellies of women.[9] But, as soon as the medical profession meddled with it, it found in it a 'foot-hold' useful to its social ascent, an application of its anatomical and pre-clinical knowledge. With professional logic it aimed at monopoly, and therefore excluded the reciprocity of services between women to replace it with a medical act, executed if possible by a duly qualified midwife, that is, by a man, a surgeon or even a doctor of medicine.

Getting to know the history of a society well, studying its social and cultural subdivisions, locating its economic cleavages, confronting the analysis of learned discourse with the facts, reconstructed patiently as with a puzzle: all these concerns, these works of detail, this taste for organising materials and questions and making them match each other, can and must save the historian from being too much himself, too much of his own time, too removed, in a word, from his ancestors, close or distant.

The analysis of sources

The sources from the proto-statistical era

Naturally, a history of health that seeks to be precise and reliable leads us to practise an analysis of sources, to gauge their limits, to focus on their vices and their faults.

The sources particular to the proto-statistical era (1770–1790) privilege the quantitative, especially in the demographic domain. This is the case in Scandinavia and in France, generally speaking.[10] What is more, it is the case for Brittany too, where the *intendants* applied the directives they received from Versailles and the ideas expressed by the Physiocrats. Their administrative zeal was stimulated by the certitude that the population of France was in decline while in fact — as we know today — it was merely experiencing a plateau. Consequently, the intendants of Brittany and their subordinates made a point of counting the population and of setting up a general register of baptisms, marriages and burials. In the same spirit, they took the greatest care to count doctors, surgeons and midwives, and to have food and medicine distributed to the 'sick poor'. This had just one purpose: to endow France with a large, particularly agricultural, population, the source of all prosperity, fiscal and military amongst other kinds. Lacking censuses, the existence of which dates from the French Revolution, the historian has other statistical material of interest at his disposal. He can file it and map it, and compare the results drawn from local monographs with the data provided by the archives of the royal Administration in Brittany or those of the Royal Society of Medicine.

Advantages and limits of the sources consulted

The historian may well ask himself if these aids were appreciated or not, if they were effective, in view of the rates of mortality that have been calculated. He may even venture into bolder hypotheses, as to whether the alliance formed at that period between the State and Medicine did not succeed that between the State and the Church, and whether a certian laicisation of knowledge about the body did not follow from this.

Two types of archival source of considerable interest present themselves. The first type has to do with mortality. The areas of deficit (in the balance of baptisms against burials) can be located year after year and placed on a chart; the designations of illnesses can be translated into modern terms whenever mentioned. Thus, the course taken by epidemics can be established at the provincial level.[11]

Better still, the second type of archives, the medical, allows us to give a name to the crises that affected the population and stimulated the royal administration to send it assistance. At the level of a group of parishes, the itinerary of the doctor, if not always of the epidemic itself, can be mapped and placed in relation to, for example, the network of roads, the great pilgrimages, the flow of travellers.

A second particular advantage of the socio-medical sources is that the historian can detect the mechanisms — social and cultural — that are the basis of the assistance provided by the State. The parish draws up the list of the 'sick poor' and asks the doctor to pay them a visit. The doctor designated by the sub-delegate arrives and examines some of the sick after enquiring into the medical topography of the locality. He then draws up a report and prescribes treatment. Next, he instructs a surgeon to go and look after the sick and gives him the list the priest had given him. Fees, travelling, medicines and alimentary assistance are at the charge of the *intendance* of Brittany.

The parish priest, though unpaid, is thus the ally of the political and administrative power; and, on different grounds (viz. the fees paid), the scientist and the 'nurse' ('soigneur') participate in the steady march of assistance, for the greater glory of a King who is the 'father of the peoples' and for the might of the kingdom. None the less, such archives are far from telling us everything, and often caricature reality, for example by identifying the quack with the swindler, thief or highway robber. The motive of such a vivid anger in the medical profession is that some 'quacks' have thrown away prescribed medicines, recommending in their place more 'popular' remedies to their clients!

In the second place, these administrative archives reveal only the medical network implanted in Brittany. Counting the number of quacks — there was a multitude of them — was never dreamed of! That is why we know only very little about the everyday life of the sick, at least in the eighteenth century. Self-medication, old wives' remedies, neighbourly help, devotional practices, pilgrimages to springs, standing stones, the tomb or the relics of saints appear only very rarely. The same goes for important characters such as the bone-setter, the village healer (*miège*), the redresser, the empiric, the wizard. Studies of a folkloric and then ethonographic character for the 18th century are lacking too, even if 'the savage' is no longer an Indian, but, sometimes a Breton peasant . . .

For all these reasons, the researcher armed with patience must investigate private archives. They alone permit us to reconstitute the life of the surgeon and the doctor, when he has left us an account book or a notebook, to know that he carried out an average of four or five medical acts a day, that his clients were not only town dwellers and that the rich often paid less well than the poor. Similarly, the exploitation of memoirs and journals, generally written by persons of quality, is absolutely necessary. The same holds true for the notes about the education of young children, their illnesses, problems with menstruation, the doctor's visits, letters addressed by the sick to their doctor — qualitative documents by any standards and all the more precious given that they are far from plentiful and that their interpretation poses difficulties.[12]

In short, if the history of mortality and morbidity can be practised positively, starting with the archives of a quantitative type produced by the administration, this does not cast any doubt, in my opinion, on the fact that a 'counter-balance' is more necessary than ever: Robert Mandrou was quite right to insist on the importance of popular literature and to make a list of the family record-books that have been preserved.[13] If one wants to understand from within the complexity of a sensibility, be it of an individual, a group or an epoch, one cannot but go beyond the approximations that the science of the 'sanitary level' provides us with and to envisage the analysis, in all its nuances, of the suffering body. To do this, it would be advisable to have recourse to the 'Bible' of French ethnologists, the work of Arnold van Gennep; but also, one should have present to one's mind the archives and/or books written by Marcel Mauss, Lucien Febvre, Claude Lévi-Strauss and, more recently, by Françoise Loux and Jean-Pierre Peter.

Methodological difficulties

The central difficulty that the historian comes up against, with the *Ancien Régime* in particular, is that there was neither actor nor spectator of the scenes he is reconstituting. What is at stake in his profession is also to tell the story, by achieving a coherent picture of the scenes he presents, working from the archival and printed material he has assembled and criticised.

More precisely, the problems the researcher meets with when he studies public health in Brittany 20 years before the Revolution are of several orders: some have to do with the diversity of the country, consisting of the normal dichotomies (sacred/profane, rural/urban, scientific/popular, illness/health) and in specific ones (Celtic/Roman, pagan/Christian, sea/land . . .). To see more clearly into all this, the historian needs to be guided by the light cast by the notions, concepts and methods worked out by different types of 'specialists': historical demographers, historians of the life sciences and historical anthropologists.

Difficulties of a demographic order

Brittany at that time consisted of around 1600 parishes divided into 65 subdelegations, and formed a généralité under the administrative direction of an intendant and of the 'States of Brittany'. It possessed about 2.2 million inhabitants, of whom a part (in the east) spoke French and the other part Breton. The majority were of Celtic culture and more or less Christianised. A Western peninsula of Europe, Brittany projects into the sea on three sides. Its climate, its soils, its economic and military activities and its epidemics all showed the effects of this, particularly at the time of the Seven Years War and of the American War.[14]

To appreciate the diversity of this great province in demographic terms, I had at my disposal while concluding this research (in the spring of 1972) two kinds of measure:

1. About twenty parochial monographs of historical demography, with the reconstitution of families, almost exclusively
   from Haute-Bretagne, that is the eastern part of the province,
   the most 'Frenchified' and hence the least 'original'.
2. Most fortunately, the inquiry ordered by the *abbé* and
   contrôleur-général Terray (between 1770 and 1787), and the
   counts undertaken at Turgot's order in 1774–5, concerned, in
   the first case, the whole of the province, and in the others,
   some interesting samples.

The apparent course taken by baptisms and burials could thus
be mapped, subdelegation by subdelegation, and even, for 1772,
parish by parish. In fact, these statistics appear relatively reliable.
The protestant minorities were minuscule in number in Brittany,
and those who died at sea were counted. However, the exiles
(though there were few of them), the floating population and the
still-born escaped the eye of the administration as they have,
massively, that of the historian. In the second place, the errors of
calculation that I was able to find in re-doing general or partial
additions are minimal. They are of the order of 1 to 5 per cent and
principally involve figures of ones or tens. Finally, they principally
affect the three first years of the inquiry, which, ordered in 1772,
goes back to 1770.

On prudential grounds, the population under study for the purpose of calculating the 'apparent' rate of mortality has been
estimated not at the level of the parish but of the regions
(subdelegations, generally speaking). Indeed, in the absence of
censuses, one is forced to use a coefficient (26 to 27) applied to a
pluri-annual average of baptisms. Pertinent on the level of the
entire province, this kind of calculation is to be treated with caution when one goes down to the level of the group of parishes, and
local crises of mortality and other events interfere.

Another important demographic problem in the sanitary situation of Brittany concerns the respective importance of crises of
subsistence and epidemics. Crises of subsistence affected only the
poorest populations, who found it hard to fill the gap between two
harvests or else those forced by high prices to eat foods dangerous
to their health such as green or ergotic rye. Even if the period from
1770 to 1790 stood outside the times of plagues and cholera, the
'epidemic diseases' as they were then called, bore the greatest
responsibility for excessive mortality in Brittany: not only the

habitual smallpox with its regular cycles, but also and especially a virulent epidemic of bacillary dysentery that spread in 1779 not only through Brittany but through the whole of the west of France.[15] Nor should one forget the epidemic of exanthematic typhus that was imported from the American Colonies by the Royal Navy in 1758.

Without a doubt, for the poorest and the abandoned a deficient and unbalanced diet facilitated the undermining of health by transmissible disease, particularly in the countryside in the interior of Brittany. It isn't an accident that twice between 1770 and 1789 crises of subsistence and epidemics coincided. Deprivation, unemployment, the lack of cash to pay for remedies and medicines (supposing they were effective anyway) created a vicious circle found today in certain under-developed countries. Infectious illnesses, which today are harmless, ravaged fragile organisms such as young children, pregnant women and the old. They also fostered the development of fatal complications for many others, when pulmonary tuberculosis, for instance, endemic in many rural areas, revived in hard times. In a country where the principal cereals (rye and buckwheat) were slow growing, because their quality depended on autumn heat, the little ice age of the period from 1750 to 1800 played a harmful role.

To this climatic conjuncture was added the naval-military conjuncture that engendered certain epidemics along the roads of Brittany. Finally, the non-central position of Brittany with regard to the main roads and the great markets served to push it a little further into the 'circle' of depression and ill-health. In this perspective the surplus of deaths, of epidemic and frumentary crises, constituted the epiphenomena particular to an immobilist society in which only the 'urban nuclei' followed the general pattern of evolution. A society, and particularly that of Brittany at the end of the *Ancien Régime*, engenders its own kind of mortality.

The retrospective diagnosis of disease and its problems

If it is possible to *estimate* the demographic situation of Brittany at the end of the *Ancien Régime*, defining the principal diseases from which the province then suffered proves to be much more difficult. In fact, today's medical diagnosis stands — *grosso modo* — at the culmination of two 'scientific revolutions': the first, clinical and anatomo-pathological; the second, bacteriological and Pasteurian. For a century, the custom has been to pronounce a diagnosis based on aetiology. At the end of the 18th century, however, even if the recognition of certain signs reminds one a little of clinical medicine (for example, smallpox), medical diagnosis was based on a chain of symptoms that did not define, in today's terms, a morbid entity. Indeed, at the end of the 18th century one is in the presence of a medicine that, while definitely learned (*savant*) is of a pre-scientific type. Medical knowledge was tied to the tradition of Hippocrates and Galen, and reasoned according to categories that have become obsolete: the humours, the temperaments and the elements. Further, this scholarly medicine was subdivided into several streams of thought,[16] which pronounced different diagnoses and prescribed conflicting treatments. Finally, one should beware of the slippages of meaning effected by vocabulary: the cold (*rhume*), under the pen of a physician of that time, generally designated a discharge or flux, not necessarily nasal, as is the meaning of the Greek *rheuma*.[17]

At first sight barbaric, obscure and therefore ridiculous, the scholarly medicine of the end of the 18th century none the less possesses its own world view and logic. But to translate the language of yesterday into current terms one requires at least two things: a long and detailed archival source describing the disease, and a knowledge of the changes that have occurred in the medical domain over nearly two centuries. To do this, one needs time, patience and even a certain 'flair'. Finally, let us be modest:

1. The historian only rarely possesses the long and detailed descriptions that constitute his 'game', an exception being made for the reports of epidemics drawn up by doctors.
2. The retrospective diagnosis that he can make often belongs to the realm of the likely, at best that of the probable, and rarely to that of the irrefutable.

Finally, it is, of course, one thing to merely name the incriminated disease; quite another to explain its causes, its propagation, its itineraries, its impact, all of which must also be explained.

J.-P. Goubert

Popular knowledge of the body

Be that as it may, the fundamental problem has to do neither with the criticism of the sources, nor the definition of the demographic *régime*, nor the distinction between crises of subsistence and crises of epidemics, nor even the elaboration of a retrospective diagnosis of disease, which are all external to their object, the body. The fundamental problem, as I see it, lies in the co-existence of two different cultures. One is above all popular and rural, and largely dominated; the other sees itself as learned (*savant*), different, even suspicious, and it impregnates the urban milieu above all.

The first stumbling-block to avoid is that of adopting as our own the judgements of one culture by the other. To recognise their autonomy with regard to principles, even if it means seeing them functioning jointly, seems to be the only acceptable solution. Popular knowledge of the body has the particularity that it establishes multiple relations, often of a cosmological type, between the events of the body and those of nature. When the order of the world is broken, disease bursts in. To re-establish order and restore the sick person to good health, certain gestures, certain rites, certain formulae are necessary, which only certain 'intermediaries', knowers of secrets, possess: blacksmiths (masters of fire), shepherds ('readers' of the sky and the stars), old women ('rich' in their experience drawn from their past pregnancies).

Intimate knowledge of the 'great book of Nature', then, leads to there being no clear dividing-line between the different 'kingdoms': the mineral world, the vegetable world and the animal/human world. Thus, the refusal by many Breton peasants to be bled, except in spring, is not devoid of logic. Outside spring, the period of rising sap in vegetables and animal/human beings, there could be no question of depriving the body of a part of its own substance, which dries up or stagnates in winter.

It was this very logic that many 'enlightened' doctors did not understand and which they christened 'superstitions'. They used this kind of discourse and this type of exclusion all the more willingly when they practised a therapeutics that, though of scholarly origin, had become popularised. The most famous example is that of theriac. Its origin was learned, to be sure: but to the doctors of the time it seemed that it could be effective only if they prescribed it themselves! Another example, perhaps less well known, consists in the overfeeding of hospital patients. This time the origin of the practice is as much learned as popular. For lack of a 'therapeutic weapon', the common idea was to reinforce the health and the 'defence' of the patient against the 'attack' of disease.

Finally, a certain number of remedies of vegetable origin (infusions, vermifuges, syrup based on 'simples') were common to the old learned medicine and to the popular practice at the end of the 18th century. In the same way, the use of alcohols and spices, recommended for 'driving out' disease, belonged to an old fund of learned medicine, the latter being humoral and belonging to the classical tradition. But under the pen of many 'enlightened' doctors, this way of doing things was relegated to an obscure, if not obscurantist past; or else it was assimilated to dangerous popular practices.

In order to better separate the grain from the chaff, that is, 'true' medicine from 'false', doctors came to speak a language in which professionalist ideology swept away historical realities. From this perspective, learned medicine cast aside the old belief in a 'universal remedy', which henceforth was seen as 'scandalous', replacing it with a trust in 'specific remedies', which alone were capable, it claimed, of effectively combatting the different 'types' of disease.

Nevertheless, while it is true that enlightened doctors were so insistent on delineating for themselves a 'professional field' for the exercise of their art, they were aware that the medicine they practised had become far removed from the sacred medicine practised as much by sorcerers as by saints, necessary intercessors between the world of men and the forces of Nature. This is why they condemned witches who tied and untied the knot, forbidding or permitting a marriage to be made and to be fertile. For the same reason, they cast the shadow of suspicion over the 'matrons' who posed a serious challenge to midwives and surgeons, indeed to not a few doctors.

Similarly again, they could not tolerate the cult of healing saints: St Méen who cures 'madness' or St Guéry who puts an end to sterility. According to our 'good doctors', it was better to come and consult them and cast these practices of the dark ages into oblivion. Or else, at the limit, for some carefully distinguished religion from medicine, the practice of certain Christian rituals appeared admissible to them, but they contested their 'medical' efficacity. Better still, they sometimes condemned certain religious practices in the name of medicine and hygiene. Thus it was with the practice of watching over the dead, when the family circle, enlarged to include neighbours and friends, assembled to pray for a whole night by the death bed. In the same way, they protested loudly against the practice of continuing to go to Sunday Mass during an epidemic. Believing in contagion, they declared against washing diseased limbs with water, even if it were holy, and, still more, against all gatherings, which favoured the propagation of certain diseases.

At the end of the 18th century, in Brittany as in many other 'provinces' of Western Europe, there coexisted, and often clashed, three cultural strata that the historian can allow himself to distinguish for the convenience of analysis. The cosmological age sees illness as a rupture of 'the order of the world', which has to be repaired by re-establishing the normal bonds uniting the body and nature. Its therapeutic is of a sacred order and is expressed in a manner at once concrete and symbolic.

The age of dominant Christianity assimilates evil and illness; it considers that only the salvation of the soul, of which the body is but, at best, the ephemeral envelope, is of importance. The only thing that counts is the way opened by the Redemption, accompanied in countries of a Catholic tradition, by the intercession of the Virgin and the saints and by 'works'.

Finally the modern age, which begins with the time of Humanism and the epoch of the Renaissance, secularises the things of the body and of nature. Henceforth, illness arises from a natural (and not divine) disorder, which human knowledge and 'science' are capable of grasping. From then on the 'professionals' drive out sorcerers, saints and healers. The analysis of these three cultural 'strata',[18] the study of their antagonisms and of their interactions, even their recovery and their condemnation by the third stratum at the end of the eighteenth century, constitutes a goal of research. This kind of research is all the more interesting in that it goes beyond the mere estimation of the 'level of health', though this remains indispensable, and allows us to question ourselves not only about the past but about the supposed certainties of our own day and age. It is all the more difficult too in that it is more exacting and involves more risks. But it is bewitching, and allows, I think, a closer approach to the heart of that 'polysemic culture of the body' of which Françoise Loux has justifiably spoken.

Finally, the history of health is particularly exacting, especially when it concerns a French province of an ancient and 'foreign' tradition. Without doubt, it 'exacts' knowledge, or rather scraps of knowledge, in demography, medicine and anthropology. But above all it demands the nose of a hunter and the ability to pass (rapidly) from the domain of abstract ideas to that of the concrete (social traditions, suffering, disease). In short, it demands critical sense and, still more, a synthetic approach.

Notes

1. *Essai sur la mortalité en Bretagne à la fin du XVIIIe siècle, 1770–1787* (Rennes, 1964).

2. This 'Diplôme d'Etudes Supérieures' (cf. no. 1) is at the origin of my PhD thesis in modern history: *Malades et médecins en Bretagne, 1770–1790* (Paris, Klincksieck, 1974).

3. Guy Thuillier, *L'imaginaire quotidien au XIXe siècle* (Paris, Economica, 1985), 99–108.

4. Maurice Le Lannou, *Géographie de la Bretagne* (Rennes, Plihon, 1950 and 1952) (2 vols.); P. Vidal de la Blache, 'Tableau géographique de la France: Bretagne', in E. Lavisse (ed.), *Histoire de la France illustrée depuis les origines jusqu'à la Révolution*, vol. 1 (Paris, 1911), 328–38.

5. Anatole le Braz, *La légende de la mort chez les Bretons Armoricains,* (Paris, 1928) (2 vols.); Marc Leproux, *Dévotions et saints guérisseurs* (Paris, 1957); Marcelle Bouteiller, *Médecine populaire d'hier et d'aujourd'hui* (Paris, 1966); Françoise Loux, *Le corps dans la société traditionelle* (Paris, 1979).

6. On this subject, see the pitfalls pointed out by Roger Chartier, 'Cultures lumières, doléances: les Cahiers de 1789', *Revue d'histoire moderne et contemporaine, XXVIII* (Jan–March 1981).

7. As an example, see the presentation by J.-P. Goubert and D. Lorillot in *1789. Le corps médical et le changement (. . .)*, (Toulouse, Privat, 1984), 9–45.

8. On this subject, J.-P. Goubert, 'L'art de guérir. Médecine savante et médecine populaire dans la France de 1790', *Annales: E.S.C., 32*, (1977), 908–26.

9. The very fine book of Jacques Gélis, *L'arbre et le fruit. La naissance dans l'Occident moderne. XVIe–XIXe siècle* (Paris, Fayard, 1984).

10. On these problems see Arthur E. Imhof and Øivind Larsen, *Sozialgeschichte und Medizin (. . .)* (Oslo and Stuttgart, 1975).

11. For some examples see J.-P. Goubert, 'Le phénomène épidémique en Bretagne à la fin du XVIIIe siècle (1770–1787)', *Annales: E.S.C.,* (1969), 1562–88.

12. For an exploitation of this kind of document see Jacques Léonard, *Les médecins de L'Ouest au XIXe siècle* (3 vols.), (Paris-Lille, 1978).

13. Robert Mandrou, *Introduction à la France moderne. Essai de psychologie historique, 1500–1640* (Paris, Albin Michel, 1961).

14. On Brittany in the eighteenth century see the thesis of Henri Freville, *L'intendance de Bretagne*, vol. III (Rennes, Plihon, 1953). See also Jean Delumeau (ed.) *Histoire de la Bretagne* (Toulouse, Privat, 1969).

15. François Lebrun, 'Une grande épidémie en France au XVIIIe

siècle: la dysenterie de 1779', in *Sur la population française au XVIIIe et XIXe siècles. Hommage à Marcel Reinhard* (Paris, Société de Démographie Historique, 1973), 403–16.

16. On this question and its effects, see especially Othmar Keel, 'The politics of health and the institutionalisation of clinical practices in Europe in the second half of the eighteenth century', in W.F. Bynum and Roy Porter (eds.), *William Hunter and the Eighteenth-century Medical World* (Cambridge, University Press, 1985), 207–56.

17. With regard to these problems, one should read with care the essential article of J.-P. Peter, 'Malades et maladies à la fin du XVIIIe siècle', *Annales: E.S.C., 22* (1967), 711–51.

18. This analysis of three cultural 'strata', in connection with the historical anthropology of birth, was presented by Jacques Gélis at my 1982–3 seminar at the Ecole des Hautes Etudes en Science Sociales.

3

Montpellier Medical Students and the Medicalisation of 18th-Century France*

Colin Jones

'Medicalisation' has been a noun to conjure with in recent decades. In the wake of the genial insights of Michel Foucault, historians have been encouraged to view the late 18th century as inaugurating in France a long-drawn-out process by which the whole of the population was progressively integrated into 'a system of medical institutions and social norms that regulated and controlled rational and prudent health behaviour.'[1] Certainly it is clear that from the late 18th century the medical profession won a prestige that substantially defused Molièresque critiques of doctors that had existed since antiquity: the doctor was henceforward a paragon, whose love for science was matched only by his love for humanity and who was now held up for admiration rather than viewed with sarcasm or contempt.[2] Certainly we also see over much the same time-scale the development of all kinds of medical syndromes — the transformation of certain kinds of spiritual crisis into mental 'illnesses' is a classic case in point — as both individual and societal developments came to be seen through medical spectacles. The 'medicalisation' label that is used to describe and locate such processes has, however developed connotations that — to put it crudely — are both 'top-down' and

*A briefer and more closely focused version of the present article was presented at the *110e Congrès national des sociétés savantes* in Montpellier in 1985 and has appeared as 'La vie et les revendications des étudiants en médecine à Montpellier au XVIIIe siècle', *Actes du 110e Congrès national des sociétés savantes. Section d'histoire des sciences et des techniques,* tome II (1985).

My revision of the paper for publication here was done while I was visiting fellow at the Shelby Cullom Davis Center, Princeton University. I would like to thank the Center and its director, Lawrence Stone, as well as another visiting fellow, Mary Lindemann, whose unpublished seminar paper 'The medical worlds of the eighteenth century' has been of great help in this revision.

'supply-sided', and which deserve challenge on both counts. The concept is construed in a 'top-down' way in that medicalisation is seen essentially as a system of social control imposed from above, with greater or lesser success, on a population now the unwitting object of medical encadrement; and the concept is 'supply-sided' in that not only have historians neglected to consider the extent to which there was a growing demand for medical services but they have also sought measures of medicalisation in supply-sided terms, such as the growing number of doctors and the increase in available hospital capacity.

In the present paper, I would like to strike a small and modest blow for a more 'demand-oriented' account of the 'medicalisation' process, which seeks to view it not as the imposition of ready-made structures on a passive populace, but more as a dynamic and dialectical process involving changing patterns of demand as well as the provision of medical services and the fixing of medical norms. Historians of demand have to accept from the start that they are at a severe disadvantage, in that the archives of demand are precisely the archives of supply, and that it is far easier to draw the rising curve of medical graduates, for example, than to analyse the contextual factors that elicited such a development.[3] The effort does, however, seem worth making.

The vignette that I will be using to discuss the point at issue is, in essence, the history of students in the University (or Faculty)[4] of medicine of Montpellier in the 18th century. Studies of student life are rather rare and tend to be negative in tone. The university in the age of Enlightenment signally failed to live up to its lofty vocation, with the result that historians, whatever their intellectual background or historiographical school, have tended to be highly negative towards the medical faculties: Foucault is dismissive; Daniel Roche's great work on provincial academies is predicated on the assumption that intellectual dynamism lay outside the groves of academe; Jean-Pierre Goubert and Dominique Lorillot call the faculties' teaching 'deplorably theoretical'; François Lebrun notes how innovatory medical teaching had always to take place 'in the margins of the archaic faculties'; Toby Gelfand is dismissive; Donald Vess, contemptuous.[5] Yet it must be said, in spite of the chorus of disdain, that we know very little about what actually went on in France's score of medical faculties in the 18th century — with the possible exception of the Paris Faculty where, it must be admitted, precious little did.[6] The provincial universities are virtually *terra incognita* in this respect, even the ancient Faculty at Montpellier, the premier medical institution of provincial France throughout the mediaeval and early modern periods. Louis Dulieu's lifetime of research on the university has, it is true, marvellously illuminated the personal life and research findings of the most outstanding Montpellier physicians — for the 18th century, the Astrucs, the Chiracs, the Boissiers de Sauvages, the Venels, the Barthez, and so on — but it has been far less directed towards questions of the nature and quality of teaching, and even less the vagaries of student life.[7]

Montpellier's medical graduates comprised the backbone of the medical corps of provincial France in the 18th century. Probably in excess of 40 per cent of the country's doctors had graduated there.[8] The University's students constituted, then, in a very real sense, the figures through whom the process of 'medicalisation' would be wrought. The Paris Faculty might have prestige and privilege, but it produced very few graduates — and fewer still who practised outside the confines of Paris and the royal court. Some other provincial faculties — notably 'degree-mills' like Orange, Nancy and Avignon[9] — produced good numbers of graduates, but the latter had very little prestige since it was generally acknowledged that virtually anyone could purchase a degree from such institutions and that, in any case, the teaching that was there offered was defective. Very few faculties indeed, as far as one can judge, matched the breadth of the syllabus at Montpellier, where the holders of eight regius professorships dispensed a teaching programme that covered all branches of medical philosophy as well as including regular anatomical and botanical demonstrations.

Prospective young physicians seem to have found Montpellier's combination of size, breadth of syllabus and intellectual lustre an increasingly attractive one over the course of the 18th century. The number of graduates the University produced on average each year rose from about 30 to 40 down to 1730 to between 60 and 80 in the last decades of the *Ancien Régime*; while the popular anatomical and botanical demonstrations brought in crowds up to 500 strong.[10] The size of the student body formed a kind of critical mass that favoured learning. This was certainly the view of the Breton Guillaume-François Laënnec — uncle of the inventor of the stethoscope — who was a student here in the 1770s: there was 'more emulation [among students] than in other faculties . . . One has the advantage of learning while having fun.'[11] The general public too seemed seduced by the medical culture that seemed to saturate the city: it was commonly said that there were more doctors than patients in Montpellier,[12] and that babies in their cradles here spouted medical Latin. It was, Laënnec held, a prejudice on the part of the public to set so much store by a Montpellier education; but, he noted (in words that underline the drift of the present argument), 'in medicine, we hold our credit solely from the public; it's silly, I know; but it is a silliness of the public, and it is only politic for a young doctor to respect it.'[13]

Materials that allow us to examine the educational experience that the University of Montpellier offered in the 18th century are not lacking, and indeed in the space here available I can only skim over some of the most important sources. The archives of the Medical Faculty in particular are in many areas exceptionally rich, and contain a good deal of virtually untapped material on the institutional life of the University in the 18th century.[14] They may be complemented by materials from a wide variety of other sources: the public documents to be found in departmental and municipal archives,[15] academic correspondence and private note-books,[16] travel literature,[17] the almost wholly untapped source of the memoirs and souvenirs of former students; and so on. Such documentation allows us to pass beyond the glitterati of 18th-century Montpellier medicine to consider the general run of medical students who, once trained, would people the French provinces as practitioners. How, then, was the run-of-the-mill doctor of provincial France trained in the 18th century? Did his training change in the period leading down to the Revolution? In what manner, if at all, did he march to the distant drums of 'medicalisation'? And what did that 'medicalisation' mean to him?

The public reputation of Montpellier's medical students was very poor indeed. The opinion of Jean-François Imbert, Chancellor of the University, in his never-to-be written history of the University, was fairly representative: 'in all periods,' he wrote, 'the spirit of the students has been the same, that is to say, a spirit of independence and insubordination.'[19] It was hardly surprising, of course, that young men, free from parental con-straints often for the first time and usually far from their homes, should have led a life that their elders and betters felt was turbulent and given to excesses. It was memories of fun and insou-ciance that came easiest to former students remembering their years at the University, and it was such qualities that struck travellers passing through Montpellier and that the public authorities deplored. The students needed, fulminated the Governor of Languedoc in 1772, a good dose of discipline, which was absolutely essential 'for good order and for the public tranquility.'[20] The student body, agreed the subdelegate of Montpellier, was 'numerous, difficult to control and full of troublemakers.'[21] How justified were such charges? And were they the whole story?

Students followed the courses given by their eight professors each weekday in term except Wednesday, which was traditionally a day off out of respect, it was said, for Hippocrates. The course of studies lasted for three years, but in fact there were no examinations for the first two and a half years. For this period, students had only to register at the University once a term, and could even absent themselves from Montpellier for much of the time. Hence, with the exception of the last six months of their studies — when they had to work long and hard to prepare for a demanding set of written and *viva voce* examinations — most students had more than enough time for distraction and amusement. It was a system of education that the *philosophe* La Mettrie — himself a physician — castigated in his usual caustic manner:

> In Montpellier, those who are destined for medical careers are for the most part young good-for-nothings who give themselves over to dissipation and indulgence for the first two years of their studies. It is only in the third that they even begin to study, in order that they may reply to frivolous questions such as: *Quid est vita?*[22]

J.E. Gilibert, a former student of the University, was even more critical. 'The first two years pass,' he claimed, 'with most students never even opening a book.' Most spent their time 'gambling in cafés, drinking in bars or courting some *grisette*.' The lecture-halls ought by right to have been full, but in fact, according to Gilibert, they usually contained only a dozen or so students — most of whom, he adds, would certainly have been asleep.[23]

These students with time on their hands certainly knew how to amuse themselves. Besides their drinking and carousing, they were also among the more assiduous clients of Montpellier's prostitutes. Some even set up their mistresses in rented rooms — much to the displeasure of the city's *bureau de police* which concerned itself with the surveillance of morals.[24] According to J.P. Willermoz, who graduated from the University in 1761, a girl had only to be seen in the company of students to be branded 'a woman of loose morals.'[25] Students were also enthusiastic players of billiards and of the 'jeu de mail', a kind of rumbustious bowls that was played in the ditches outside the city ramparts.[26] The latter sport was witnessed in 1737 by the young Jean-Jacques Rousseau as he passed through the city. He found the medical students 'very good boys . . . less debauched than they were noisy, less licentious than gay,' and opined that 'in spite of the bad reputation of the students, I found more morality and fellow-feeling amongst those youths than could easily be found amongst the same number of fully-formed men.'[27]

A further manifestation of the students' rather carefree attitude towards their studies was their taste for fashionable clothes. The northerner Guillaume-François Laënnec felt himself utterly outclassed by the flashy attire donned by his southern colleagues during his period of study in Montpellier. Sumptuous dress-sense went in tandem, moreover, with a taste for fencing — purportedly a quintessentially 'noble' pursuit.[28] One of the first steps that the young Théophile de Bordeu, the future court physician and *philosophe*, had taken when registering as a medical student in 1739 had been to engage the services of a fencing-master.[29] Later in the century, Laënnec was to express astonishment at the 'itch for swordsplay' that was, he maintained, 'epidemical' among the students.[30] The rigorous prohibition on the wearing of arms that the University imposed at numerous junctures throughout the late 17th and 18th centuries came to be bolstered by decrees of the Governor of Languedoc who expressed his bafflement at this 'rage for fencing (among the students) which appears to me to have very little to do with the career for which they are destined.'[31] Yet his decrees had no more effect in stamping out swordsmanship than the resolutions of the faculty.

Although students often kept their swordsmanship to themselves, they also channelled their violence against two secular groups of arch-rivals. The rivalry with soldiers, who were numerous in Montpellier, which was a garrison-town, often resulted in duels, at the bottom of which one suspects rivalry for a woman.[32] Antagonism towards surgeons, on the other hand, manifested itself in a kind of guerrilla warfare. The age-old rivalry between the two groups seems to have been given added edge in the 18th century by the development of a more respectable, more intellectually progressive and more professional surgery, and medical students clearly found it difficult to accept that their erstwhile inferiors were well on the way towards becoming their equals. Throughout the century, the two groups were at daggers drawn. The University's botanical and anatomical demonstrations were on occasion disrupted by their brawling. Even when seemingly engrossed in night-time grave-digging, surgeons and students fell on one another in gang fights, before the arrival of the city watch sent them fleeing for the shadows.[33]

Turbulent, licentious, *aficionados* of individual and group violence, the medical students of Montpellier were very protective of what they claimed were their rights. The University of Montpellier was an institution with a clearly 'democratic' tradition[34] (by contrast with the more 'magisterial' universities like that of Paris), which was held to be composed of the teaching and the student bodies in their entirety. The students were very much aware that they had, and always had had, an important role in the corporative life of the University. Their chosen representatives — whose ancestors we find as far back as the 14th century, and who from 1550 were known as 'student councillors' (*conseillers des étudiants*) — were allowed to attend *ex officio* all solemn and official ceremonies of the academic year.[35] In accordance with an ancient usage — which had by the 18th century, it is true, become rather symbolic — the professors of the university were not even allowed to receive their salaries until the student councillors had attested that they had performed their teaching responsibilities satisfactorily.

A further example of student involvement in the life of the university was their participation in appointments to professorial chairs, notably during the public *viva voce* examinations (or *disputes*) of candidates by the existing faculty members. On the eve of the public session in which candidates to chairs delivered their so-called *triduane* theses, they made an official protocol visit to all the city dignitaries (the bishop of Montpellier, the Governor and Intendant of Languedoc, the First President of the *Cour des Aides,* etc.), accompanied by a crowd of students stewarded by their councillors. When the visits were over, the candidates brought the students back to the university buildings where they had laid on for them a sumptuous banquet. Following complaints from a number of professorial candidates in 1757, the central government intervened to outlaw this custom, which, it was said, was deterring potential candidates from competing for chairs because of the excessive costs and the drunkenness and debauchery that accompanied disputes. The University professors, however, protested strongly against the prohibition of a practice that they claimed was immemorial and which moreover had the salubrious effect of keeping the students quiet during the *disputes* themselves. 'Not long ago', they pointed out, 'the son of a professor claimed that as such he was immune from this obligation towards the students; he could not avoid the whistling of the students (in his part in the *dispute*) and he had to do as his competitors had done so as to keep the students quiet.'[36] The latter, for their part, seem to have taken their right to rowdiness very seriously, and continued to exercise it down to the Revolution despite the warnings of 1757.

In all this, as in much else in their collective life, the students appear to have been marshalled and led by their councillors. Selected by the professors from a shortlist submitted by the assembly of students, the four councillors were the accredited leaders of the student body. Among students elected to the post in the first half of the 18th century, we find the names of many future professors and medical luminaries.[37] To be chosen student councillor was thus, it would appear, a privilege accorded the most outstanding and intellectually precocious students. Besides their presence in university meetings, the councillors also had the right to assist as unpaid helpers in the botany demonstrations that were held each summer; and they were also held responsible for delivering to the university corpses from the city hospital, the Hôtel-Dieu Saint-Eloi, for the winter course in anatomy — a course in which they were accorded the signal right of participating in the dissections. It was, furthermore, to the student councillors that were sent free theatre tickets to which students were entitled and which they then distributed among a student body every bit as keen, it would appear, to attend a theatrical performance as an operating theatre!

The councillors had other responsibilities too, which helped ensure the cohesion, well-being and morale of the student body. They acted as a kind of welfare- and reception-committee for new arrivals to Montpellier, and according to the professor Jean Astruc, were responsible for instructing the latter 'in the usages of the University and the rules to which they were to conform.'[38] The councillors provided too for those students who fell ill or became hard-up. This indeed was a far from negligible task, for most students, whether French or from abroad, were far from their homes. The councillors acquitted themselves well in this respect, in the opinion of Chancellor Imbert, who noted: 'The councillors — as I have seen for myself — provided for sick students, with the greatest assiduity, all the help, including financial aid, that they might lack.'[39] Their role in student welfare was prophylactic too. The professor Boissier de Sauvages, in his multivolume *Nosologie*, noted of *la nostalgie*, that homesickness and pining that beset so many individuals far from home in the early modern period, that its best remedies were 'the support of friends, games, spectacles, parties, money', and went on to note that 'the students of Montpellier are rarely subject (to the condition), for they find in the company of their friends enough to compensate for the absence of their parents and, with so many ways of entertaining themselves available, they soon forget them.'[40]

A further, highly important role of the councillors was to act as liaison between the professoriate and the student body. According to Imbert, 'through the councillors, the University was kept informed of any abuses developing among the students. Through the voices of their councillors, the students communicated their demands and their complaints to the University which by this channel informed the students of its decisions.'[41]

Although the institution of councillors could thus act as a channel of communication — and perhaps as a safety-valve — the student representatives were not always popular with the faculty, who at times saw them less as 'pacifiers' than as 'trouble-makers.' This was particularly the case towards the middle of the 18th century when the students began to issue a number of demands concerning the status of the councillors and the position of the student body within the Faculty. In much the same way that feudal lawyers were at this time combing through ancient land-registers to discover seigneurial rights that had fallen into decay, the students began to scrutinise old legislative texts in order to prove that their consecrated rights were not being properly respected, and that their power in decision-making was only a shadow of what by rights it ought to have been. In 1750, increasingly aware of the grumblings of student discontent, the professoriate formally deplored 'the flames of independence and revolt' sweeping through the student body, while the latter for their part claimed that they 'formed a body apart from and independent of the University' which consequently could be

governed by different laws and customs. The situation took a turn
for the worse when the professors suspended the councillors from
their posts, claiming them to be leaders of student rebellion.
Tempers flared. Students began to insult and threaten their professors; they organised the boycotting of lectures; and they placed
pickets at the gates of the University. The rebellion was only
extinguished when the Governor of Languedoc stepped in,
imprisoning the student leaders, issuing stern admonitions against
the rest of the student body and formally abolishing the post of
student councillor.[42]

The professors restored the student councillors in 1760. They
soon regretted it. Violence and unruliness increased, student
demands redoubled, and the professors were soon deploring the
'raising of the standard of a new revolt.' The students were now,
interestingly, expressing their demands in a Montesquieu-esque
language that prefigured some of the constitutional disputes of
1789: the student body, they argued, should be viewed as 'the
house of commons, whose decisions depend on the opinion of the
upper chamber.' This new wave of student contestation was eventually broken by the professors expelling the ring-leaders and
again abolishing the post of student councillor.[43]

In 1770, the professors tried a new tack, by appointing four
'student syndics'. These were intended to have many of the more
positive and constructive aspects of the old councillors, but not the
same rights — they were not permitted, for example, to attend
university meetings and ceremonies.[44] Perhaps as a result, the
syndics do not seem to have achieved the same level of support
from their fellow students as the councillors had done. In 1772,
Laënnec — in a metaphor that evidently came easily to a medical
student — commented regretfully on how the corporative
organisation of the students 'was today no more than a
dismembered skeleton which each day is being progressively
carved up.'[45] Another revealing sign of the times was the vogue
that freemasonary came to enjoy among the students. Did the
students abandon their former organisations for the masonic
lodges in much the same way that the mediterranean bourgeoisie
was transferring their allegiance, from *confréries des penitents* to
masonic lodges, as Maurice Agulhon has shown?[46] Certainly, the
lodges provided much of the welfare support that the student
councillors had formerly organised. The *Coeurs Réunis* lodge,
established in 1781, was composed very largely of students and
young doctors (along with, significantly, a fencing-master), and its

officials proudly proclaimed that 'it was virtually for the University that [the lodge] had been established, and it was by the University that it would be for ever perpetuated.'[47]

It could be argued that the picture I have painted so far of an agitated and unruly student body and of a professoriate that with greater or lesser success strove to get them to toe the line is neither unusual nor even necessarily specific to the 18th century. Indeed it is tempting to collapse these picturesque episodes — which aptly bear out the poor reputation of Montpellier students that I mentioned earlier — into the *longue durée*, not to say into the timelessness, of academic life. However, I would like to go from here to argue that, if we examine their contestation closely, we can see that many students in fact took their studies very seriously indeed, and that by means of demands, petitions, classroom unruliness and the occasional bout of direct action they had in their sights not only the structure of the University but also the very nature and content of medical education therein offered. Students were in fact attacking an education that they found increasingly defective, overly theoretical and insufficiently grounded in practical studies.

One of the prime targets of the students was the poor quality of the teaching they were given, and in particular the number of professors who did not fulfil their teaching responsibilities properly. In 1728, the students petitioned the Chancellor of France, complaining that several of their professors gave no classes at all, that others only gave a few, and that not all branches of medicine were covered in the university syllabus. One of the professors, Henri Haguenot, supported their case — thus winning for himself the enduring hostility of his colleagues — remarking that 'most professors, some because they have more lucrative occupations, others because they do not like their job, totally neglect their responsibilities, and in particular the giving of public lecture-courses.'[48]

Despite a severe reprimand from the Chancellor of France, the professoriate seems not to have mended its ways appreciably. In 1738, the Montpellier students drew up a new petition. Anatomy classes were petering out after only a fortnight. As for the botanical demonstrations, 'the first five or six are ordinarily all right, but the others are conducted with extraordinary haste and with a marked distaste on the part of the professor.' One professor had not given any classes at all for two years, another for a very long time on grounds of the weather ('in winter he excuses himself on account of the cold, in summer on account of the heat'). Another professor never appeared in person in the lecture-hall, preferring to send his son in his place to read out his father's lecture notes . . .[49]

It was much the same story still in 1739. The students this time were particularly severe on the university's Chancellor, Jean-François Chicoyneau, who, it was claimed, 'prefers to get himself drunk on wine and to see his mistresses rather than to teach us.'[50] From the 1760s, a new rash of criticisms occurred. The students' complaints centred increasingly on *subrogation*, that is, the practice of a professor using a replacement to give his courses for him. In 1778, for example, a doctor from the city who was deputising for the great vitalist Pierre-Joseph Barthez during one of the latter's frequent absences from Montpellier had his classes boycotted by all medical students and was reduced to lecturing before a hall composed solely of apprentice surgeons.[51]

The professors rebutted many of the students' complaints as excessive and ill-founded. *Subrogation* did at least show that classes were taking place properly. It was, moreover, they argued, a necessary evil, in that they were often called away to provide treatment for persons of distinction. By maintaining a numerous and well-connected clientele, they kept intact the reputation that the Montpellier faculty had always had of being skilful practitioners, at the same time that they supplemented their excessively low university stipends (the level of most of which had been set in the 16th century). Were they to be prevented from attending to the health of their wealthy clients, they argued — even if the latter were located far away from Montpellier — then the quality of the teaching that the professors provided would be irremediably damaged, and the lustre of the faculty severely tarnished.[52]

The professors utilised a similar kind of argument to defend their practice of giving private lessons — a practice that was often viciously attacked by students over the last decades of the *Ancien Régime*.[53] The students saw in such fee-paying courses a rather dubious commerce that devalued the public lecture courses and increased the cost of medical education. The professors, in contrast, maintained that only such supplements to their pitifully low salaries kept them in the job. They also pointed out that private courses given to a small elite of students were the prime means of instruction in all the top medical schools of Enlightenment Europe (Vienna, Leyden, Edinburgh, etc.). It was, they argued, by small-group teaching rather than by Latinate harangues before half-empty amphitheatres, that the best teaching was done — and in particular in regard to clinical or practical medicine.[54]

Practical medicine: this was indeed one of the slogans of student contestation throughout the last half-century of the *Ancien Régime*. Far from viewing their studies solely with a frivolous eye, many students took their education seriously enough to demand insistently an improvement in the teaching of practical aspects of medicine. Since 1715, in fact, the *pensum* of one of the holders of Montpellier's eight professorial chairs had been the treatment of the sick poor.[55] But the chair had never functioned in this way. Moreover, the administrators of Montpellier's main hospital, the Hôtel-Dieu Saint-Eloi, had always resisted the attempted incursions of the professors into the medical service of the hospital for they feared them prioritising research and teaching over accommodating the susceptibilities of the sick poor within hospital walls.[56] Such an attitude had serious consequences for students wishing to engage in practical aspects of the medical art.

Students had for a long time been in the habit of visiting the Hôtel-Dieu Saint-Eloi in the company of the institution's doctor, an individual who normally did not teach at the University. In 1746, this custom was formally recognised by the hospital's administrative board, which did in return, however, insist that the students should conduct themselves with reticence and decency in the presence of the sick poor.[57] The students appear to have found the administration's restrictions something of a strait-jacket, and in 1760 they petitioned the administrative board to complain of the speed with which the hospital doctor conducted his rounds, and the lack of consideration he showed towards medical students who were accompanying him. The hospital administrators came down on the side of their doctor, and became even more stringent as regards the presence and conduct of the students. The latter were henceforward to comport themselves 'in the greatest silence and with the greatest modesty,' and were to 'avoid tiring the sick by too many questions regarding the state of weakness or exhaustion in which they find themselves.'[58] In 1783, similar considerations of decency appear to have been operative in leading the hospital board to forbid medical students to enter the female wards.[59]

Student discontent seems to have tailed off somewhat in the last years of the *Ancien Régime*. This may have been partly due to the popular courses on practical medicine and therapeutics that several professors — including Barthez when he was there — started to give, and partly also due to the teaching visits that the University Chancellor Imbert succeeded in establishing from 1769 in the Hôpital Saint-Louis in Montpellier, a military hospital that admitted soldiers with venereal and cutaneous diseases.[60] Chaptal, Napoleon's Minister of the Interior under the Consulate, would remember having been struck, on registering in the faculty in 1774, by the extent to which 'practical medicine was everything.'[61] The students continued moreover to concern themselves with the efficacity of the teaching that was provided for them. In 1772 and 1773 they issued petitions calling on the University to finance a demonstrator to teach them the most popular pharmaceutical preparations.[62] In 1782 and 1783 they combined with the professors to request the central government to accord them a grant that would allow them to create a medical library.[63] They also made insistent demands for the refurbishing of the university's botanical gardens, which were falling into disrepair.[64]

In the final analysis, it seems fair to conclude that the rather grim picture of university life in 18th-century Montpellier painted by many contemporaries was somewhat exaggerated. The students — and who would be surprised by this? — were often gross, sometimes frivolous and occasionally turbulent. But the other side of the coin was that a great many students were serious, studious and indeed enthusiastic for a form of medical education that was less theoretical and more biased towards practical experience than had hitherto been available. The early careers of a number of notable Montpellier graduates illustrate this more pronounced thirst for medical practice. Théophile de Bordeu, for example, studied in Montpellier between 1739 and 1746. Though he graduated in 1742, he remained in the city, giving private anatomy courses, even though occasionally he was obliged to substitute for human corpses the mortal remains of the city's stray dogs! Significantly, he had no qualms about getting involved in the traditional domain of the surgeons, nor about consulting with the leading surgeons of the city.[65] A similar open-mindedness was demonstrated by the young Pierre-Joseph Willermoz, who lodged with a surgeon, whom he accompanied on his rounds, before registering as a medical student in 1759. He too would maintain good relations with the city's surgeons, and would foster close relations as well with the local apothecaries.[66] The young Pierre Bourquenod is another interesting case-history. The son of one of the city's leading surgical dynasties, he served as apprentice-surgeon at the Hôtel-Dieu Saint-Eloi, a wonderful theatre for surgical experience, but withdrew from the hospital in 1763 to inscribe at the Faculty.[67] In earlier times, the fact that he had practised the 'mechanical' arts of surgery would have been sufficient to disbar him from a university education. But now the University closed its eyes to such precedents. Indeed, sensitive takers of the public's pulse (metaphorically as well as literally), the professors encouraged a greater open-mindedness between the different branches of the medical profession. In 1728, for example, the University had created a 'doctorate in surgery', which experienced a greater popularity from the 1760s onwards.[68]

I have endeavoured thus far to establish that Montpellier's medical students in the 18th century were in the vanguard of attempts to modernise medical teaching by introducing a much stronger practical component into their education. Why did they do so? One might be tempted to see their attitude in terms of ideological osmosis. Certainly, their professors shared much of their distrust of a system of education that could result in a student graduating as a doctor without ever being at the bedside of a sick person, and were in their different ways aware of the slow but inexorable shift taking place from a medicine grounded in the texts of Antiquity to a more scientifically based, empirically oriented medicine. Many doubtless too would feel part of the broader current of ideas that prized the practical, the useful, as the *summum bonum*. Some of this probably did rub off on the students. But how much? Perhaps it is safer to speculate that the general run of students were motivated less by scientific than by career considerations: that is, that students believed that an education more heavily grounded in practical medicine would stand them in better stead for their careers once they had obtained their doctorates.

What is certain — and this would seem to fit in neatly with a 'demand-side' explanation for the phenomenon under consideration — is that newly qualified doctors would have to find a clientele among a public far more choosy and better-informed on medical questions than in the past. In particular, anatomy, dissections and surgical operations became a kind of vogue among the general public everywhere. 'Knowledge of anatomy is of concern to all men,' declared the *Encyclopédie* orotundly.[69] In Montpellier, as elsewhere, fashionable folk frequented dissection theatres in their droves. Surgical intervention was also highly popular: indeed the nurses at the Hôtel-Dieu Saint-Eloi complained that the poor inmates were being trampled on in their beds by the crowds of students and sightseers who came to witness operations in the main wards, and these complaints led in fact to the creation of a separate operating theatre with full accommodation for viewing.[70] With a public like this — so enthusiastically wedded to the fashion for anatomical knowledge — to gain their living from, many students would surely have felt that they needed to know more about anatomy than the traditional medical course had offered. Strong public demand also helps to explain why Montpellier's innovatory 'doctorate in surgery' was such a resounding success. One can better understand too certain other, perhaps excessive, reactions on the part of students: the penchant for grave-robbing, for example, resulted less (one assumes!) from necrophilia than from a desire to perfect anatomical knowledge in the best way available.

The general public's growing interest in things anatomical and surgical seems to have been part of a broader shift in *mentalités* regarding life and death. The decline in the 18th century of the old mortality crises that, sparked by war, famine, epidemic disease or a combination of these, had insistently afflicted French society, seems to have produced something of a lightening of the intellectual and emotional atmosphere. If among the poor — as the classic work of Olwen Hufton has clearly demonstrated[71] — matters of life, death, disease and subsistence retained much of their gloomy cogency, among the upper and middle classes at very least, the grim reaper cast a less threatening shadow. Historians have often argued that the decline in mortality crises helped to trigger a 'dechristianisation' of attitudes in French society generally.[72] I would suggest that another, perhaps partly overlapping, feature of the change in *mentalités* was a growing concern for health. As cosmological explanations lost ground to materialistic and mechanistic ones, disease was seen less in terms of God's punishment, more as the product of faulty bodily functioning. Faulty, moreover, and often remediable malfunctioning, for the changed views of health put a higher rating on preservation than on resigned acceptance. Symptomatically, *la médecine préservatrice* was viewed as one of the keys to human progress in that intellectual testament to Enlightenment optimism Condorcet's *Esquisse d'un tableau historique des progrès de l'esprit humain.*[73]

One consequence of the growing middle- and upper-class concern with health and its preservation was that many areas of life became more heavily charged with positive medical values —

more 'medicalised,' if one likes. Changing *mentalités* among their putative clientele also meant that the medical profession could view itself increasingly as the technicians of the booming new culture of health maintenance.[74] This was a heady transformation, and among many medical practitioners it elicited a more flexible and interventionistic approach, and a greater sensitivity to the presentation of their medical services. 'Medicine is a commodity that everyone wants,' quipped La Mettrie.[75] Medical historians have in the past been perhaps too willing to write off the *philosophe*-physician as a throwback to Molière, but in the light of the present argument it would be more appropriate to view him as a prophet of the new trend of medical commercialism. Doctors were in essence nothing but 'merchants in medicine,' 'kinds of traders who all go hunting for gold and silver, though by different and circuitous routes.'[76] Medicine was in essence only a branch of rhetoric: what the patient wanted to hear was always the key consideration, in persuading him to part with his money in exchange for the medical 'commodity' of health.

Perhaps because they have not been willing enough to consider the changing pattern and volume of demand for medical services, perhaps too because they have too often taken at face value doctors' own estimates of their motivation as disinterested and above sordid monetary considerations, medical historians have consistently undervalued developments in 18th-century medicine that bespeak a commercial approach to medicine and a greater sensitivity to the market for their services. Even the Mesmerist cult — perhaps the most striking illustration of the new cult of health and well-being — is often written off as an example of man's constant ability to be duped, rather than analysed as a classic case-study in medical entrepreneurship.[77] The growth of medical journalism and, in particular, medical advertising and self-publicity, are other features of the medical scene that have not been fully appreciated.[78] The emergence of private mad-houses — not as widespread in France as in England, it is true, for many monasteries were still willing to accept lunatics on presentation of a royal *lettre de cachet* — is another development in which doctors could amass fortunes: the career of asylum-manager Jacques Belhomme, for example, is a most illuminating illustration of medical 'playing-to-the-market.'[79] Similar examples could doubtless be found in the world of mineral spas and compound remedies.[80] The efficacy of treatment for venereal disease knew no great breakthrough in the 18th century: yet the constantly changing pattern of provision for individuals afflicted with syphilis and gonorrhoea is a further — and most regrettably ill-researched — example of medical entrepreneurship.[81] When set against this veritable jungle of opportunism and sensitivity to the market, the activities of Montpellier's medical students, in agitating for a course that would prepare them for the attitudes and prejudices of their potential clients, becomes instantly more comprehensible. As Guillaume-François Laënnec had noted, it was 'only politic' for young physicians to respect public prejudices.

Changing attitudes towards health made the 18th century a golden era of medical opportunity. Conditions were made strained, even cut-throat, however, by the fact that doctors were competing for public custom not only with each other but with a range of other practitioners. Prominent among these were the pot-pourri of non-licenced practitioners — wise-women, religious communities of nurses, travelling bone-setters and dentists, local wizards and so on — whom the doctors branded as 'charlatans.'[82] The whole campaign to outlaw charlatanism in the late 18th and early 19th centuries, which historians once saw as a gauge of the self-assurance of the medical profession, is now more realistically viewed as a gesture of desperation to try to keep potential clients away from rival practitioners.[83] (And particularly threatening rivals at that, since the 'charlatans' were often better known, more trusted and cheaper than the practitioners of 'establishment' medicine, as well as being more adept at playing to the gallery, for much medical charlatanism shaded imperceptibly into something akin to show-business.)[86]

Even more worrying for the 18th-century medical graduate, moreover, was competition from the quarter of the surgeons. The ancient demarcation line between doctors and surgeons was wearing thin in the 18th century, as surgeons abandoned their traditional inferiority complex and became enterprising, autonomous and increasingly 'professionalised' in their conduct.[85] Surgeons became fashionable with upper- and middle-class patients, especially in regard to three very well remunerated specialties: venereal disease (in theory an 'external' illness, and their province rather than that of the 'internalist' doctor); childbirth (the surgeon-cum-male-midwife was coming to replace the gross *matrone* at the bedsides of women of the middle and upper classes); and inoculation against smallpox (the fashionableness of which was crowned by the royal family's adoption of the practice from the late 1750s).[86] Such was the success of the surgeons in winning the confidence of their patrons, moreover, that doctors even ended up imitating them in several respects. Certainly, the success of Montpellier University's 'doctorate in surgery' and the students' calls for more anatomically and surgically based instruction witness the extent to which the doctors felt that the old ways were not enough. It was not that society was passively surrendering to the schemes of 'medicalisation' offered by a self-confident medical profession: there was a demand for 'medicalisation' on the public's own terms, which doctors, surgeons, charlatans, and even Montpellier's medical students, in their very different ways, were trying to satisfy.

Notes

Place of publication is Paris for works in French unless otherwise stated.

1. M. Foucault, *Surveiller et punir: naissance de la prison* (1975; English translation as *Discipline and punish: the birth of the prison*, New York, 1976), p. 135. Foucault's work has been very influential in popularising the term 'medicalisation.' See his *Folie et déraison. Histoire de la folie à l'âge classique* (1961; abbreviated English translation as *Madness and civilisation: a history of insanity in the age of reason*, New York, 1965); *Naissance de la clinique: une archéologie du regard médical* (1963: English translation as *The Birth of the clinic*, London, 1974); and (with others) *Les machines à guérir (aux origines de l'hôpital moderne)* (1976).

A good introduction to how the term has been handled by French historians working more within the tradition of the *Annales* school is J.-P. Goubert, 'La médicalisation de la société française à la fin du XVIIIe siècle', *Francia, 8* (1980). Special issues of journals devoted to the topic include *Annales. Economies. Sociétés. Civilisations, 32* (1977) ('Médecins, médecine et société en France aux XVIIe et XVIIIe siècles': much of which has been translated as R. Forster and O. Ranum (eds.), *Medicine and society in France. Selections from the Annales* (Baltimore and London, 1980); 'La médicalisation en France du XVIIIe au début du XXe siècle', *Annales de Bretagne, 86* (1979), and, 'La médicalisation de la société française, 1770–1830', *Réflexions historiques/Historical Reflections, 9* (1982). At a general level too, see the collective work *Médecins, climat et épidémies à la fin du XVIIIe siècle* (1972: especially the article by J.P. Peter); and J. Léonard, *La France médicale: médecins et malades au XIXe siècle* (1978). Regional theses that contribute to the debate include F. Lebrun, *Les hommes et la mort en Anjou aux XVIIe et XVIIIe siècles. Essai de démographie et psychologie historiques* (1971); J.-P. Goubert, *Malades et médecins en Bretagne, 1770–1790* (1974); G. Frêche, *Toulouse et la région Midi-Pyrénées au siècle des Lumières* (1976); and P.L. Thillaud, *Les maladies et la médecine en pays Basque nord à la fin de l'Ancien Régime (1680–1789)* (Geneva, 1983). See too J.-P. Goubert and F. Lebrun, 'Médecins et chirurgiens dans la société française du XVIIIe siècle', *Annales Cisalpines d'histoire sociale, 4* (1973); F. Loux, 'Recours convergent à la médecine officielle et à la médecine parallèle en matière de soins aux enfants en France (XIXe–XXe siècles)', in A.E. Imhof (ed.) *Mensch und Gesundheit in der Geschichte* (Husum, 1980); and G.D. Sussman, 'Enlightened health reform, professional medicine and traditional society: the cantonal physicians of the Bas-Rhin, 1810–70', *Bulletin of the history of medicine, 51* (1977).

2. An introduction to the tradition of anti-medical satire is be found in C.J. Witkowski, *Les Médecins au théâtre de l'antiquité au XVIIe siècle* (1905). For the changing image of the physician in the 18th century, G. Chaussinand-Nogaret, 'Nobles médecins et médecins de cour au XVIIIe siècle', and D. Roche, 'Talents, raison et sacrifice: l'image du médecin des Lumières d'après les Eloges de la Société royale de Médecine (1776–1789)', both in *Annales. Economies. Sociétés . Civilisations, 32* (1977). The article by Roche is available in English translation as 'Talent, reason, sacrifice: the physician during the Enlightenment', in Forster and Ranum (eds.), *Medicine and society in France*.

3. For some data on medical graduates, M. Compère, R. Chartier and D. Julia, *L'Education en France du XVIe au XVIIIe siècle* (1976), p. 273–4. For comment and case studies of 'demand-centred' history, see N. McKendrick (ed.), *The birth of a consumer society: the commercialization of eighteenth-century England* (Bloomington, Indiana, 1982).

4. Either term is acceptable, as in some respects the institution was the medical faculty of the University of Montpellier, and in others the University of Medicine of Montpellier. For an introduction to the university's history in the 18th century, A. Germain, 'L'Ecole de médecine de Montpellier. Ses origines, sa constitution, son enseignement', *Mémoires de la Société archéologique de Montpellier, vii* (1877–81); and L. Dulieu, *La Médecine à Montpellier. 3. L'époque classique. Première partie* (1983).

5. Michel Foucault's views on the sterility of 18th century medicine are well known (see especially his *Birth of the clinic*); D. Roche, *Le Siècle des Lumières en province: académies et académiciens provinciaux, 1680–1789* (1978); J.-P. Goubert and D. Lorillot, *Les cahiers de doléances des médecins, chirurgiens et apothicaires. 1789, le corps médical et le changement* (Toulouse, 1984), p. 15; F. Lebrun, *Se soigner autrefois. Médecins, saints et sorciers aux XVIIe et XVIIIe siècles* (1983), p. 37; T. Gelfand, *Professionalising modern medicine. Paris surgeons and medical science and institutions in the eighteenth century* (Greenwood Press, Westport, Connecticut, 1980); D. Vess, *Medical Revolution in France, 1789–96* (Florida University Press, Gainesville, Florida, 1974).

6. Besides Gelfand's work cited in the previous note, see M. Staum, *Cabanis. Enlightenment and medical philosophy in the French revolution* (Princeton, New Jersey, 1980), 95–101; and A. Corlieu, *L'ancienne Faculté de médecine de Paris* (1877).

7. L. Dulieu, *La Médecine à Montpellier*, 3. We await the appearance of the second volume of this study for a full bibliography, including Dr Dulieu's own extremely extensive writings.

8. According to statistics compiled in the early years of the 19th century, 1101 of 2530 physicians practising in France who had been trained prior to 1789 had graduated from Montpellier. M.E. Antoine and

J. Waquet, 'La médecine civile à l'époque napoléonienne et le legs du XVIIIe siècle', *Revue de l'Institut Napoléon*, no. 132 (1976).

9. F. Lebrun, *Se soigner autrefois*, 27–37.

10. M. Compère *et al.*, *L'Education en France*, 270–1 for a graph, based on the archives of the Faculty of Medicine, S 23–54.

11. A. Rouxeau, *Un Etudiant en médecine quimperois (Guillaume-François Laënnec) aux derniers jours de l'Ancien Régime (1768–74)* (Nantes, 1926).

12. The city's population was about 30,000!

13. A. Rouxeau, *Un Etudiant en médecine quimperois*.

14. A printed inventory of the archives of the Faculty of Medicine (henceforth = AFM) exists: *Cartulaire de l'Université de Montpellier. Tome II, deuxième partie. Inventaire numerique des archives anciennes de la Faculté de Médecine* (Montpellier, 1912). The archives are located in the library of the Faculty, Rue de l'Evêché, Montpellier, which also includes many valuable printed materials concerning the life of the Faculty. Pride of place among these, from the point of view of the students, must go to the baccalaureate theses, which exist in their hundreds for the 18th century and which have never been systematically exploited.

15. The Archives Départmentales de l'Hérault (henceforth = ADH) contain relevant materials in series C (Intendance of Languedoc — especially related to public order problems), series G (secular clergy — material relating in particular to the bishop of Montpellier who was formally Chancellor of the University of Montpellier), and series D (learned societies). The municipal archives of Montpellier also contain much of interest, notably series FF (municipal police).

16. Examples of correspondence are the Willermoz and Haguenot papers, cited below in notes 25 and 48. There are likely to be similar collections in archival depots throughout France and indeed Europe at large, given the wide range of localities from which Montpellier students hailed. Archives and libraries can also be expected to contain student notebooks of dictated notes and other materials. For an excellent example, see the notebooks of the Montpellier student, then professor, Boissier de Sauvages, ADH 10 F 51, 53.

17. Large numbers of tourists passed through or stayed in the city in the 18th century. For some English examples, see M. Sacquin, 'Les Anglais à Montpellier et à Nice pendant la deuxième moitié du siècle', *Dix-huitième Siècle, 13* (1981). See too, below, note 27.

18. One has to know where to look. Gilibert's memoirs of his student days (see below, note 23) are to be found, very thinly disguised, in a basically theoretical work. See notes 23 and 61 below.

19. AFM C 91.

20. AFM F 57.

21. ADH C 88.

22. J. Offray de la Mettrie, *Ouvrage de Penelope, ou Machiavel en médecine*, vol. 2 (Berlin, 1748–50), 257.

23. J.E. Gilibert, *L'Anarchie médicinale, ou la Médecine considérée comme nuisible à la société* (Neuchâtel, 1772), 36–9.

24. Archives municipales de Montpellier, FF (unclassified registers of the bureau de police). For Montpellier's world of prostitution, C. Jones, 'Prostitution and the ruling class in eighteenth-century Montpellier,'

History Workshop, 6 (1978).

25. Bibliothèque municipale de Lyon, ms 5525 bis: Willermoz correspondence.

26. 'Montpellier en 1768, d'après un manuscrit anonyme inedit,' in J. Berthelé, *Archives de la ville de Montpellier. Inventaires et documents,* vol. 4, 52–3, 151, 157.

27. J.-J. Rousseau, *Confessions* (Pléiade edition, 1959), 258.

28. ADH C 525. See Bibliothèque municipale de Montpellier, ms 590.

29. Théophile de Bordeu, in M. Fletcher (ed.), *Correspondance,* vol. 1 (Pau, 1973), 37.

30. A. Rouxeau, *Un Etudiant en médecine quimperois,* 87.

31. ADH C 525. For prohibitions on the carrying of arms, etc.: AFM C 48 (1678), C 57 (1740), ADH C 530 (1757), AFM C 60 (1760), ADH C 525 (1766), G 1321 (1767).

32. ADH C 88, AFM C 74, F 52, F 53, Q 104.

33. AFM S 16, S 63, ADH C 524, etc.

34. See A. Cobban, 'Medieval student power', *Past and Present,* no. 53 (1971); and A. Germain, *Du principe démocratique dans les anciennes Ecoles de Montpellier* (Montpellier, 1881).

35. See esp. AFM C 91, an important memorandum in the hand of Chancellor Imbert, on the institution of student councillors and on student representation and organisation generally.

36. ADH C 529; AFM D 70. Cf. the picturesque details of the *dispute* of 1790 in (R.D. Dufriche des Genettes), *Souvenirs de la fin du XVIIIe siècle et du commencement du XIXe siècle, ou Mémoires de RDG* (2 vols., 1835–6), vol. 2

37. For example: Marcot (1701), H. Haguenot and Fizes (1706), F. Chicoyneau (1722), Venel (1741), Imbert (1745), Broussonet (1751) . . . For details about the student councillors, see esp. AFM C 91.

38. J. Astruc, *Mémoires pour servir à l'histoire de la Faculté de Médecine de Montpellier* (1767), 78.

39. AFM C 91.

40. F. de Boissier de Sauvages, *Nosologie méthodique,* vol. 7 (Lyon, 1772), 239–40.

41. AFM C 91.

42. For this whole episode: ADH C 529, AFM C 88, C 91, F 41. See too ADH C 6786.

43. AFM C 90, C 91. See too AFM C 65, F 48, S 26, S 17; and ADH G 1320.

44. AFM C 91.

45. A. Rouxeau, *Un Etudiant en médecine quimperois,* 85.

46. M. Agulhon, *Pénitents et francs-maçons de l'ancienne Provence* (1968); and, more specifically on Montpellier, G. Laurans, 'Contribution à l'étude sociologique des confréries de pénitents en Bas Languedoc,' unpublished *thèse de troisième cycle,* Sociology, (Montpellier, 1973).

47. Bibliothèque Nationale FM (2) 310–14; ADH 1 J 11; AFM S 124. See A. Germain, 'Une loge maçonnique d'étudiants à Montpellier', *Académie des Sciences et Lettres de Montpellier. Section des Lettres* (1876–80).

48. ADH C 529; and Archives anciennes de l'Hôtel-Dieu de Montpellier (henceforth = HD), B 90, B 93.

49. ADH C 529.

50. Ibid.

51. AFM D 94, Q 163, S 17, S 127; ADH G 1322. See, for *subrogation*, ADH G 1320.

52. ADH C 524, C 530.

53. ADH C 524; AFM C 91.

54. See the comment of F. Lebrun, *Se soigner autrefois*, 57.

55. L. Dulieu, *La Médecine à Montpellier*, 3.

56. For a general discussion of this point, C. Jones, *Charity and 'bienfaisance': the treatment of the poor in the Montpellier region, 1740–1815* (Cambridge, 1982), 124–8.

57. ADH HD B 87.

58. ADH HD E 8.

59. ADH HD E 12.

60. ADH C 555.

61. J.C. Chaptal, *Mes souvenirs sur Napoléon* (1893), p. 16.

62. AFM C 76, C 77.

63. AFM F 68, Q 159.

64. ADH G 1322; AFM Q 27.

65. Biographical material on Bordeu in his *Correspondance*, vol. 1, passim.

66. Willermoz correspondence (reference in note 25 above).

67. ADH HD E 9.

68. AFM Q 53, S 18; and L. Dulieu, 'Pierre Chirac: sa vie, ses écrits, ses idées', *Montpellier médical* (1957).

69. Cited in P. Ariès, *L'Homme devant la mort* (1977), 359. And, for women, see the highly anecdotal, but interesting A. Cabanès, 'Les femmes du monde aux cours de médecine' in his *Moeurs intimes du passé*, 5th series, esp. p. 311 ff.

70. ADH HD E 9.

71. O. Hufton, *The Poor of eighteenth-century France, 1750–89* (Oxford, 1974).

72. For introductions to the burgeoning literature on 'dechristianisation,' see M. Vovelle, *Piété baroque et déchristianisation au XVIIIe siècle: les attitudes devant la mort d'après les clauses des testaments* (1977); and J. Delumeau, 'Au sujet de la déchristianisation', *Revue d'histoire moderne et contemporaine, 22* (1975). See too J. McManners, *Death and the Enlightenment. Changing attitudes to death among christians and unbelievers in eighteenth-century France* (Oxford, 1981), esp. pp. 440–5.

73. Condorcet, in O.H. Prior (ed.), *Esquisse d'un tableau historique des progrès de l'esprit humain* (1933), 236.

74. Cf. the convergent arguments of M. Foucault in his *Histoire de la sexualité. I. La volonté de savoir* (1976).

75. La Mettrie, *Ouvrage de Penelope*.

76. La Mettrie, *Ouvrage de Penelope*.

77. Though see R. Darnton, *Mesmerism and the end of the Enlightenment in France* (Cambridge, Mass., 1968).

78. For an English example of the medical juice to be squeezed from periodical literature, R. Porter, 'Lay medical knowledge in the eighteenth century: the evidence of the "Gentleman's Magazine"', *Medical History*,

32 (1984). For France, cf. E. Wickersheimer, *Index chronologique des périodiques médicaux de la France, 1679–1856* (1910); and R. Taton (ed.) *Enseignement et diffusion des sciences en France au XVIIIe siècle* (1964), 216–18, 222–3, etc.

79. On Belhomme, the anecdotal G. Lenôtre, *Paris révolutionnaire. Vieilles maisons, vieux and papiers*, 3rd series (1921) is useful; and on *lettres de cachet*, see A. Farge and M. Foucault, *Le Désordre des familles: lettres de cachet des archives de la Bastille au XVIIIe siècle* (1982).

80. See F. Lebrun, *Se soigner autrefois*, 79–82. On this, as on many other neglected aspects of medical 'consumption,' of great use is P. Delaunay, *Le Monde médical parisien au XVIIIe siècle* (1906).

81. There are some wonderful studies on venereal disease waiting to be written by those with strong stomachs: the archival and printed materials are excellent. See P. Delaunay, *Le Monde médical parisien*, for a sampler.

82. J.-P. Goubert, 'The art of healing: learned medicine and popular medicine in the France of 1790', in Forster and Ranum (eds.), *Medicine and society in France;* T. Gelfand, 'Medical professionals and charlatans: the Comité de Salubrité *enquête* of 1790–1,' *Histoire sociale/Social History, 11* (1978).

83. See esp. J. Léonard, 'Women, religion and medicine', in Forster and Ranum (eds.), *Medicine and society in France;* M. Ramsay, 'Medical power and popular medicine: illegal healers in 19th century France', *Journal of Social History, 10* (1977); and M. Ramsay, 'Sous le régime de la législation de 1801: trois enquêtes sur les charlatans au XIXe siècle,' *Revue d'histoire moderne et contemporaine, 7* (1980) and J. Leonard, 'Les guérisseurs en France au XIXe siècle,' ibid.

84. See C. Jones, *Charity and 'bienfaisance'*, 117–18.

85. T. Gelfand, *Professionalising modern medicine*, is the key source here.

86. The correspondence of the Montpellier medical faculty is full of complaints from rural practitioners concerning the manoeuvrings of the surgical profession: AFM, esp. series F. For midwifery, see M. Laget, *Naissances. L'accouchement avant l'âge de la clinique* (1982); M. Laget 'Childbirth in seventeenth- and eighteenth-century France: obstetrical practices and collective attitudes', in Forster and Ranum (eds.), *Medicine and society in France*; and J. Gélis, 'Sages-femmes et accoucheurs: l'obstétrique populaire aux XVIIe et XVIIIe siècles', *Annales: E.S.C., 32* (1977).

4

Popular Culture and Knowledge of the Body: Infancy and the Medical Anthropologist*

Françoise Loux

The position of researchers in one discipline is a difficult one to maintain within a debate internal to another discipline, especially when questions of methodology are at issue and sister disciplines, such as history and anthropology, are involved. For my part, the best way to handle it is doubtless to take my own discipline as a starting point and to analyse from that basis the points of convergence, of divergence, and of over-lap with other disciplines. I think, moreover, that if one wants to avoid being trapped within an endless theoretical debate over the relation between anthropology and history, discussions must of necessity proceed on the basis of concrete research.

That is what I hope to do by showing how, in the course of my own research on the body and on infancy, I found myself brushing shoulders with historians working on related problems and how I became aware of both the specificity and the relatedness of our respective methods.

Indeed, in a great many areas — the body is undoubtedly a particularly revealing instance of this — French historians and ethnologists are working more and more closely together and are thus preparing the ground for a common historical anthropology, This necessary complementarity must not, however, mask the specificity of either approach, which, in my view, is more often than not more a matter of nuances, of over-all orientation, than of very sharp distinctions.

In France, this complementarity is a rather recent phenomenon. This is not the place to trace back the history of the

---

* Translated by Sylvana Tomaselli

developments of these disciplines. Let us just recall that ethnology won its spurs in 'exotic' societies, all too readily deemed static, and in which history isn't, therefore, an essential factor. For a long time ethnology in France had the academically inferior and rather disregarded status of folklore, of the study of traditions related to a vague, nebulous past. It is not surprising, therefore, that relations with historians were only tenuous and that the latter were long rather doubtful of folklorists' observations, thinking that they lacked rigour.

There have, none the less, been some exceptions to this. Let us cite — on the side of history — the essential work of Marc Bloch, *The Royal Touch.*[1] On the side of folklore, the writings of P. Nourry-Saintyves are still all too little known.[2] Despite their apparent evolutionist and positivist aspects, his books, rich as they are in fascinating lines of future research on symbolism and the imaginary, await rediscovery. He constantly has recourse to history, especially that of the Middle-Ages, and he often draws on the work of historians such as Jean-Claude Schmitt[3] and Jacques Gélis.[4] It is obviously not incidental that the work of Saintyves bears largely on the body and medicine. Indeed, as soon as one begins to be interested in popular medicine, one quickly realises that it is difficult to study it without reference to learned medicine, especially that of the Mediaeval and Renaissance periods.[5] This quite naturally leads one into history.

In work devoid of Saintyves' rigour, however, this research into origins often has a confused, quasi-mythical, character that has little explanatory force. This has therefore led ethnologists to insist, until quite recently, on the internal coherence and meaning of this popular medicine, whatever its origins, which, in turn, led them almost inevitably to neglect a historical approach.[6] That is what Claude Lévi-Strauss has often been accused of by those who misconstrue him. In his final analysis, he was particularly clear on this point. It isn't a matter of societies with or without history, but of societies that 'frankly' own up to their historical character, considering it 'as a tool to act on the present and to transform it', and of others that 'are hostile to it and prefer to ignore it', considering it 'as a disorder and a threat'.[7]

It remains none the less true that at the level of practice numerous ethnologists have kept their distance from history, a distance doubtless necessary to the constitution of their discipline. Paradoxically this has been all the more necessary in the case of complex European societies, impregnated with history, because it was necessary to ascertain that, despite the inter-relations and the phenomena of power and dominance, there existed a popular culture, less directly discernible in texts than in the recesses of discourses, of testimonies, and through oral documents. This demonstration is now all but complete, and a new reconciliation has been brought about between historians and ethnologists. Ethnologists have begun to be less neglectful of the social and temporal dimensions of the phenomena they were studying, while historians have become more sensitive to anthropological notions such as those of symbolism and internal coherence. The work of Carlo Ginzburg[8] and Jean-Pierre Peter[9] has, in my opinion, been crucial to this development. Indeed both emphasise the need to analyse the 'hollows' within official discourse. Whether we consider the discourse pertaining to the repression of the Benedattis or of Menocchio in Ginzburg's work, or the flaws within physicians's discourse in Jean-Pierre Peter's work[9], something else emerges through which one can discern a little of the reality of what was being attacked: popular wisdoms (savoirs), beliefs and practices. In some recent books, it is becoming difficult to distinguish what pertains to history and what to anthropology. Let us cite, for instance, the research of Marie-Christine Pouchelle, analysing, as an anthropologist, the representations of the body by a mediaeval surgeon, Henri de Mondeville.[5] She locates very precisely the surgeon's work both in relation to the medical movements and the ideas of the period, while also teasing out the symbolic representations of the body through a painstaking analysis of all the book's metaphors. When the historian Jacques Gélis wants, on the other hand, to study the considerable changes that attended birth between the 16th and the 18th centuries, he deems it essential to undertake first and foremost an anthropology of birth,[4] analysing this phenomenon within the wider framework of symbolic relations between man's body, nature and the cosmos — still a widely held representation in 19th century traditional France, brought to light by the folklorists on whose work Jacques Gélis constantly draws.

However, the two disciplines, although mutually drawing on one another, have none the less maintained a certain specificity: the anthropologist remains in spite of everything more sensitive to non-variable factors and to symbolisms; the historian is more concerned to analyse variations and perhaps also relations to institutions.

This is not the occasion for me to draw the balance sheet of the state of research in France from this angle in the last few years. What I would like to do instead is to list a number of both theoretical and methodological problems occurring at the juncture between the two disciplines. But first, let me begin with the data of my own research to make myself clearer.

My research on popular culture and the body

Before I start, however, let me just say a few words about the overall framework of this research. I have been engaged in this project for some 15 years at the Centre d'Ethnologie Française, a laboratory located in the Musée National des Arts et Traditions populaires. It bears essentially on the body and its meaning in French rural society towards the end of the 19th century.

On the basis of specific examples taken in particular from the domain of infancy, I have tried to show that there existed a culture, a set of traditional knowledge pertaining to the body, with its own coherence and mode of transmission, which, however, doesn't imply that it is completely independent from learned culture. It is this internal coherence that has caught my attention in my research into the general signification of the body (especially through proverbs), in my research on infancy and the meaning of teething, as well as in my current research on the content of popular medical recipes. I have also analysed the transmission of knowledge pertaining to the body and nature in research still in progress on mountain guides (not the books but the humans).

Finally, I am interested in the complex problem of the relation between learned and popular as revealed through two research projects: one, just mentioned, on recipes in popular medicine; the other on chap-books, and, more generally, on the literature popularising medical advice and recipes in the 18th and 19th centuries.

Within this entire field of research, a certain amount of material and methods represents, in my view, non-variable factors. I would like to insist on three points. First, I have conducted a specific research project on proverbs,[9] but I also use them a great deal through the rest of my research. It is often said that there is a paucity of material on traditional rural life. But in actual fact, provided one knows how to interpret it and, especially, provided one doesn't confuse discourse and practice, there is more material available than is generally thought. Thus all proverbs pertaining to physicians are hostile. One shouldn't infer from this that peasants, familar with these proverbs, were therefore necessarily hostile to physicians themselves. What we are dealing with in this instance is a discourse, and it is incumbent on us to find the reasons that led to so aggressive a discourse as well as its function.

Proverbs make up a body of very rich material, gathered by folklorists towards the end of the 19th century. Provided one doesn't use this kind of source uncritically, which isn't very difficult, proverbs may be considered as direct records of what was being said and thought about the body in rural society while they were common currency.

Secondly, the material on which I have worked is often historically specific on two counts. On the one hand, it would be possible to think in terms of origins, to find a given proverb in a literary work, for instance; such wasn't my particular concern. It was sufficient for me that two given proverbs, even of different origins, occurred at the same time. In this respect my procedure was not that of a historian. On the other hand, my reading of French rural society towards the end of the 19th century has of course, been a reading of that time in its own right (and in this respect it comes near to that of a historian), but it was also based on the underlying assumption that this would allow a better comprehension and understanding of our present society. It is with this in mind that I work with various health experts, to reflect on the relation between these traditions and present health care.[11] This may come down to saying that I want to reflect on our own anchoring into the past, on our historical roots. Once again, this perspective shows the ethnologist rather than the historian in me. The distance that classical ethnologists place between their society and the exotic society they study is introduced in my case by the temporal dimension.[12]

Thirdly, what all these pieces of research have in common is the constant recourse to field-work, less to systematically compare the traditional with the contemporary than to verify, to vivify, certain hypotheses. Thus it is from the standpoint of a bookish knowledge of traditional beliefs that I was able to understand that expectant mothers' refusals to weigh themselves, which I observed in my field-work, wasn't a matter of carelessness, but a preventive practice. Besides, the persistence of certain practices, even when physicians advise against them, which I observed on the field, helped me better to understand a similar attitude that I encountered in my literary data. Field-work enriches my archival work and vice versa, without there always being a direct relation, a continuity, between them. I would even go so far as to venture that there cannot be a one-to-one relation between materials of too different a nature. Yet this confrontation with the field seems indispensable to me.

Problems regarding a critical use of sources and of the contextualisation of these sources also occur at the level of material accumulated during field-work, especially in relation to the context of the investigation. The experience I have gained working on folklorists' materials as well as through being critical of the manner in which these have been gathered, without always locating them precisely in the social context of their utterances, enables me sometimes to be more rigorous in my approach when I return to the field. It often takes several meetings before getting beyond the polite vacuities of the first encounters. However, the vagueness of some of the recollections also has a meaning. Thus terms such as 'always', 'in the olden days' are always meaningless for a historian; for an anthropologist they must be interpreted in terms of attitudes to the past; if, for instance, it is claimed that something has always been known, what is thereby indicated is that this knowledge is so old that it constitutes one's identity. Even in cases in which the dating is mistaken, discovering the reasons and the functions of this 'mistake' is meaningful for the anthropologist.

In all aspects, my research is therefore close to historical research bearing on the same social categories and the same period, but it none the less has its own specific character.

Let us now turn to more detailed examples.

Research on infancy

My research on the specific theme of the care of the young child's body, undertaken some ten years ago, had a double starting point. First, my previous research on the body had demonstrated the central role played by infancy: proverbs often refer to it, therapeutic rituals often focus on it. There is nothing surprising about this: it is a period in life that was, on the one hand, particularly vulnerable, and on the other, essential to the transmission of knowledge pertaining to the body.

Secondly, there was a further question, which the work of demographic historians raised for me. At the time when I undertook this research, the issue of infant mortality and its relation to putting children out to nurse was indeed a prominent one. The rather hasty conclusion had been drawn that the practices of wet-nurses and, more generally, of country women were dangerous, owing either to their indifference, or to a more-or-less conscious desire for infanticide; and it was believed that they contributed significantly to infant mortality. My intention is not — nor has it ever been — to discuss the complex nexus of problems related to the use of wet-nurses, either from the point of the parents or from that of the wet-nurse.[13] Nor was it a matter of unqualifyingly denying indifference, neglect, much less infanticide, in one single sweep. The problem I set myself was rather whether the examples generally given as instances of negligent behaviour on the part of the mothers — such as that of the dirtiness of children's hair — could genuinely be considered as such. I was hampered by an ethnocentric assumption, that of folklorists and physicians of the 18th century and, more especially of the 19th century, which consisted in isolating a practice and judging it according to our own norms.

Before drawing any kind of conclusion, it thus seems necessary to analyse the practices of mothers in their entirety and to see how each individual practice takes on, or fails to take on, a meaning in relation to other practices.

I often compare my undertaking to doing a puzzle in that I place all the elements in relation to one another to see in what way an ultimate coherence is, or isn't, generated. I will give only one example of this.[14]

The dirtiness of children, and especially of their hair, is generally taken as an example of negligence on the part of the parents. A great number of things may be said on this subject. They may be summarised as follows: first, washing a child inside a rural interior, exposed to draughts, is to risk his catching cold. Now cold was particularly feared for frail people — the old, the ill, children — in rural society. Leaving them dirty was therefore preferred to exposing them to this risk. Secondly, it had especially to do with the head — hence a selective kind of dirtiness. In fact, the child's head was the object of particular attention because, being the seat of the brain and intelligence, it was one of the signs of the humanity that infants acquired by degree. Now the fontanelle was a particular cause for concern. On the one hand, it was one of the signs of the incompleteness of the child; on the other, the child's brain seemed particularly vulnerable on account of it. It was thought to be quite permeable — as, for example, from too vigorous a soaping — and also easily penetrated. It was feared that worms might penetrate into the brain through the fontanelle, causing meningitis, or that draughts might cause a fatal inflammation of the brain.

For all these reasons, the dirtiness of the head was regarded as a protective layer — a second skin — coming to reinforce the fontanelle.

Besides, in this society, the body's wastes, as they symbolised the body in its entirety, could not be disposed of in any casual way. On the one hand, they could be used for witchcraft; on the other, the disappearance of a part of the body prefigured that of the whole, that is death. This is made evident, for instance, in the restrictions bearing on washing clothes.

Here it is obvious that not to wash a child, or rather, to wash him but little, constituted a protective practice. I say, to wash him but little, because, in this society, one must also be aware of nuances: what, from our present perspective, seems like a state of real filthiness, admitted of fundamental nuances ranging from negligence to preventive practice.

What I have tried to demonstrate with this example is that it isn't enough to prove, even with the aid of statistics, that some practices are harmful, to establish that they were intentionally so. The intention can only be grasped from within, by analysing the meaning of those practices.

Research on popular medical knowledge

In the course of my research on the body in traditional France I have often come across chap-books: almanacs containing proverbs, books of medical recipes, books on health care. Morever, amongst historians and literary specialists, there has been an extensive debate about the readership of these chap-books: popular literature, for or against the people.[15] My conclusions, in the limited field of booklets bearing on the body are consistent with those of other researchers such as Lise Andriès.[16] With respect to their origins, these booklets are all more-or-less directly derived from learned works. However, the finer details of analysis and comparison between texts show that at the beginning these simplfied editions were not conceived with a popular readership in mind. It is only in the 19th century that entire booklets specifically aimed at this readership begin to appear. But even in these pamphlets it seems that there was not a complete overlap between recipes from popular medicine — such as those collected by folklorists — and medical recipes such as those disseminated by almanacs.

This research brought me to consider, at the borderline with history, questions of the reinterpretation and absorption of text in relation to its own culture, of the relation between the oral and the written. Now this kind of research can proceed only on the basis of concrete and exact material. It is on this level in my opinion, that the quantitative intervenes. I have thus undertaken some research on the whole body of French recipes of popular medicine gathered together by folklorists at the end of the 19th century. This research has several intended aims: first, to constitute a corpus accessible in due course to the whole of the scientific community; secondly, to draw up an inventory of the illnesses mentioned and the ingredients used; thirdly, to analyse the place they occupy within a series of rituals linking the concrete to the symbolic; finally, to analyse their relations to advice disseminated by chap-books.

It is in fact only by starting from a quantitative analysis that we will be able to move ahead in the analysis of the relations between learned and popular, by shedding light on precise questions of reinterpretation, copying and innovation. However, this quantitative analysis will only yield hypotheses, leading once again to qualitative research. In my opinion, all research proceeds in this manner, oscillating constantly between qualitative and quantitative. In the current phase of this research, I underline the qualitative aspect. Indeed, my colleague, the computer scientist P. Richard, and I have begun to set up a very detailed coding system enabling us to take into account all the aspects of the recipe: material, but also ritual aspects too (such as saying a prayer, making the sign of the cross, or using an intermediary to which one transfers the illness). This precise coding could only be carried out by myself and, in any case, it was necessarily rather reductionist and artificial. The first results we have obtained are interesting, but show that our pre-established analytical categories (illnesses and therapeutic ingredients) are not very revealing, and must be broken down into elements (symptoms, properties of the ingredients, gestures) that acquire meaning only when assembled, not into fixed groupings but into relational networks. Infections, for instance, are related both to the category of humours and to that of inflammations.

One of the questions that currently concerns us in relation to this research is the following: shouldn't we keep the computer, in such a case, for adding, drawing up inventories (of illnesses, ingredients . . .) and simple correlations (between illnesses and plants, for instance), and leave more precise research on the same corpus, everything requiring a complex analysis (such as prayers for healing or the use of ritual gestures) to be done 'by hand'?

Anthropology and history, two complementary approaches

After this somewhat general presentation of my work, it seems appropriate to take up again, in a more synthetic manner, problems that anthropology and history clearly have in common.

Permanence and variation

One of the more persistent debates is that of the relative importance each discipline grants to permanence and variation.

The historian, like the sociologist, tends to be more interested in what is specific to a period, a social class, what distinguishes them. Whether it is in the long term or not, he tries to spot periods of transition, of rupture. In contrast, the anthropologist is more concerned with what Lévi-Strauss calls the non-variable, that is, with continuity, with what endures or persists in a new form under change.

This represents in my view two different but complementary forms of approach to social change. Thus, the anthropologist interested in non-variables is concerned to show that changes, ruptures, are never radical, that they are preceded by slow slidings. His contribution may help nuance the evolutions that historians sometimes describe a little too much from the outside. In the case of the ethnologist, the almost complete absence of interest in duration, in dating, may lead to some imprecisions. In this case, contact with history is particularly rewarding, at least as far as ethnology in France is concerned, in that it forces one to be precise and even to put into question, once again, the all-too-nebulous notions of tradition, of traditional society.

The fact remains that in spite of changes, the non-variable elements are always far more numerous than one would think at first glance; it is anthropology's great contribution to have brought them to light. For instance, where the historian only sees the absence of maternal love or interest in the child, an anthropologist analyses an interest made manifest in different ways. But within the context of his own research, any researcher can only shift from one method to the other: how could one be interested in the non-variable without having been first concerned to highlight the particular tone of each culture. Besides, beyond permanence — once this permanence is emphasised — it may well be that one should again be concerned with the diversity of each particular tone. Thus, taking up the example of the dirtiness of infants once again, the constant factor is the relation between the state of cleanliness of the body and prevention; the specific coloration or tone is the dirtiness for traditional rural society and the extreme cleanliness of our own period.

Function and content

Another point of divergence between approaches that none the less remain complementary overall is, in my opinion, that of function and content, well illustrated, for instance, in the French edition of Carlo Ginzburg's book, *The Night Battles*, by a discussion between the author, Daniel Fabre and Giordana Charuty about the work of Jeanne Favret on witchcraft.[8]

There are, indeed, two possible ways of approaching a discourse or a practice. Either one approaches it in relation to the function that it plays within society; one thus analyses its social variations, its historical changes. Such is the method most frequently adopted by historians as well as by sociologists. In contrast, ethnologists are more likely to analyse the internal coherence of a given culture by entering it. All too often, these types of analyses, that of function and that of content, have been opposed to one another to such an extent that some, such as Jeanne Favret, consider the content of objects, of the symbolic forms being used as insignificant objects when they are analysing, with otherwise great accuracy, witchcraft proceedings.[17] Similarly, for Dan Sperber,[18] the symbol is inconsequential to the form of the objects on which it is materialised. By contrast, Carlo Ginzburg shows the great merit of a study taking content for its basis — as that of confessions in witchcraft trials.[8]

What is interesting is that this bringing together of content and function, or this opposition, occurred within the disciplines themselves — some historians wanting to go beyond the simple notion of function while some ethnologists were questioning the inclusion of an analysis of content.

In my opinion, there is once again complementarity rather than opposition between function and content. With respect to rituals, for instance, their prophylactic function in relation to anxiety or their function of perpetuation of power is essential, but the detailed analysis of the phases of these rituals and the elements they put into play is equally essential to the realisation of these functions.

At the level of popular medicine, for instance, the function of the healer within society comes into play in relation to the efficacy of the remedy. An artisan or peasant is like the sick people he attends to; he gives the latter the right to be ill or reintegrates him or her into society. But the remedies that he gives must also be carefully analysed: the anti-inflammatory properties of such a plant or such a colour or shape recalling the ailing part of the body (for instance, the dentated leaves of ferns are good for toothaches).

All this contributes to giving, or failing to give, one or several meanings to illness, to inserting it within society and culture.[19] Research can dispense with neither one, nor the other, aspect, yet owing to their training and the tendencies within their disciplines, sociologists and historians will tend to privilege the first approach and ethnologists the second. In any case, analysis of the content of material such as rituals is far from having revealed all there is to be said about the functioning of society. Jeanne Favret shows, for instance, on the basis of a detailed comparison between elements involved in rituals of bewitchment (the colours of the cards, the sharpness of the objects . . .), the function of the 'trigger of violence' in these rituals, which leads to a precise analysis of social relations in villages.

Symbolism and empiricism

One of the undeniable contributions of anthropology is the emphasis it places on the symbolic dimension. An approach in functional terms often has the tendency to privilege the technical dimension (this is efficacious . . . this isn't) especially with regards to medicine and the body whereas history has had the tendency to present itself only in terms of progress. But it isn't the case that just because a practice is inefficacious in our eyes it has always been so, and that is where the notion of symbolic efficaciousness, of correspondence to a given system comes in. For instance, the 'grand-mothers' who relieve the pains from burns, in a given context, by blowing on the burn while muttering a prayer, have an unquestionable efficacity for persons who believe in it and who feel themselves to be in tune with the gestures made and the words uttered.

Generally, in popular medicine, practices must be analysed at two separate levels constantly interpenetrated: the practical level no less than the symbolic level. If one doesn't take this second level into account, one tends to consider everything that doesn't fit into the framework of provable efficaciousness as 'superstition'.

Thus, Mireille Laget has just published an important book, presenting an analysis of Dom Nicholas Alexandre's medicine for the poor,[20] in which, with the aid of a pharmacologist, she offers an explanation for these recipes, either in relation to the medical theories of the period, or, what is more interesting still, in terms of modern theories close to homeopathy. Such an in-depth study had never before been undertaken, and it constitutes a fundamental work in history for many reasons. However, a more anthropological approach, one that would analyse more directly the symbolism of the ingredients employed by this medicine and which would thereby reveal more completely its rationality and coherence, should complement this research. This would require the drawing up of a list of all the therapeutic ingredients used, relating them to the illnesses, and seeing whether any constants, such as the correlation of the colour yellow with urine or the colour red with blood, emerge.

Coherence and divergent logic

Another familiar feature of anthropology is its emphasis on the fact that there are different types of rationality and logic. Similarly, it has been shown that the term 'superstition' is often an ethnocentric manner of speaking about beliefs one doesn't share.

From this point of view, the historical approach and the ethnological can also diverge. Because of the areas it investigates, the historical approach tends to take on the perspective of society taken in its entirety and studies popular culture in relation to it. There is hence a tendency to speak, as in sociology, of dominant culture, to analyse phenomena in terms of origins and, often, to consider that popular culture is made of obsolete residues of scientific culture. The anthropological approach — on account of its experience of exotic terrains — has instead more of a tendency to start from the internal coherence of a culture, and not to be too concerned with an analysis in terms of origins, but to see how all the elements are integrated or contradict one another. It then establishes a coherence, if such a coherence exists for the members of the culture in question, without worrying about the diversity of origins of the various elements. In my work on proverbs, for instance, I was able to show that all proverbs, however diverse their origins, were interrelated through the themes of death and of the relation between health and work, and thus that proverbial discourse pertaining to the body has a deep-seated coherence. Similarly, the recipes of popular medicine often came from old learned medicine, but they have been transformed, reinterpreted, by the addition of gestures, formulae, through the precision of a number, of a colour, which tend to stress the symbolic aspect.

There again, the two approaches are complementary. But history may well have forced ethnology to be more rigorous in its appreciation of this coherence, by underlining the fact that the elements are often disparate and, especially, that one mustn't forget the relations of force and power that regularly oppose dominant to dominated culture. Ethnology quite simply first taught the historian to admit of the existence of a relatively autonomous popular culture, then to analyse it.

Rigour

This leads me to conclude on the subject of rigour. The fact that history and anthropology are social sciences leads too often to an insistence on method and the requisite rigour. This sometimes consists in hiding behind this method.

Recourse to the computer can sometimes be an instance of this. I have often had to give advice to research apprentices for whom the quantitative was a refuge against the absence of hypotheses.

I think — and the important influence within French ethnology of authors such as Michel Leiris[21] is obviously very marked in this context — that social sciences, if they want to remain productive, cannot and should not be sciences entirely like the others. Especially in matters of the history and anthropology of medicine, one must be wary of being too easily influenced by medical scientific approaches, which, as it happens, are often receptive to quantitative approaches.

I think that one must insist a great deal — and this isn't done sufficiently — on intuition, floating observation, such as Colette Petonnet describes it, in relation to urban anthropology taking, for example, the Parisian cemetery, Le Père Lachaise.[22] She spends long periods of time, at different times of the day, wandering through it, looking at the graves, speaking to strangers; thereby without her really deciding to do it, the lines of force of the terrain construct themselves gradually within her. At the beginning of a piece of research, a long, necessarily vague, period seems essential. This doesn't preclude rigour in the gathering and critique of material, nor even the intervention of the quantitative and the computer. I don't think there is any cause to make sharp demarcations between these two aspects. But as the most rewarding research of these last years shows, the qualitative plays an important and significant role in all valuable research.

Notes

1. Marc Bloch, *Les rois thaumaturges* (Paris, Gallimard, 1986) with an introduction by J. Le Goff.

2. See for instance, *L'astrologie populaire, et l'influence de la lune* (Paris, Nourry, 1937); *En marge de la légende dorée: Songes, miracles et survivances* (Paris, Nourry, 1930); *Les saints successeurs des Dieux* (Paris, Nourry, 1907).

3. Jean-Claude Schmitt, *The Holy Greyhound: Guinefort, healer of children since the thirteenth century*, trans. Martin Thom (Cambridge, 1983).

4. Jacques Gélis, *L'arbre et le fruit: la naissance dans l'occident moderne XVIe–XIXe siècle* (Paris, Fayard, 1984).

5. See in particular the very illuminating notations in M.-C. Pouchelle, *Corps et chirurgie à l'apogée du Moyen-Age,* (Flammarion , 1984).

6. My own work on the body certainly has this characteristic in so far as it insists on the internal coherence of popular knowledge: see more especially *Le corps dans la société traditionnelle* (Paris, Berger-Levrault, 1978) and *L'Ogre et la dent* (Paris, Berger-Levrault, 1979).

7. Claude Lévi-Strauss, 'Histoire et ethnologie', *Annales, 11–12* (1983), 1217–31.

8. C. Ginzburg, *Le fromage et les vers. L'univers d'un meunier du 16e siècle.* trad. française (Flammarion, 1980); *Les batailles nocturnes: sorcellerie et rituels agraires dans le Frioul, 16e et 17e siècles* (trad. française) (Verdier, 1980).

9. Following the seminal article by Jean-Pierre Peter and Jacques Revel, 'Le corps. L'homme malade et son histoire' in *Faire de l'histoire* (Gallimard, 1974), a number of ethnologists and historians met regularly at Jean-Pierre Peter's seminars on the body; that is how real exchanges between researchers from the two disciplines came about, as between Marie-France Morel and myself: 'L'enfance et les savoirs sur le corps.

Pratiques medicinales et pratiques populaires dans la France tradition-nelle'. *Ethnologie Fran*çaise, 3–4, (1976) 309–24. Jean-Pierre Peter is without a doubt amongst the first historians to have realised the necessity of 'another' reading of texts, highlighting, through the hollows of the discourse, a hidden or denied reality. He was also one of the first to have insisted on the anthropological approach and on the search for a discourse's or a cultural practice's own internal coherence. See in particular, 'Entre femmes et médecins. Violence et singularités dans les discours du corps et sur le corps d'après les manuscrits médicaux de la fin du 18e siècle', *Ethnologie française, 3–4* (1976), 341–8, and 'L'histoire par les oreilles, Notes sur l'assertion et le fait dans la médecine des lumières', *Le temps de la reflexion* (Gallimard, 1980), 293–319.

10. Françoise Loux and Philippe Richard, *Sagesse du corps, Santé et maladie dans les proverbes réginaux français* (Maisonneuve et Larose, 1978).

11. Françoise Loux, *Tradition et soins d'aujourd'hui* (Interédition, 1983).

12. The use of this method is especially well illustrated by the recent work of two sociologists, who, in order to show the recent changes within representations of illness and the ill find it necessary to produce a vast historical perspective; Claudine Herzlich and Janine Pierret, *Malades d'hier, malades d'aujourd'hui* (Payot, 1984).

13. On this subject see, Fanny Fay-Salloy, *Les nourrices à Paris au XIXe siècle* (Payot, 1980); Jacques Gélis, Mireille Laget and Marie-France Morel, *Entrer dans la vie* (Gallimard, Coll. Archives, 1978).

14. For greater detail, see F. Loux, *Le jeune enfant et son corps dans la médecine traditionelle* (Flammarion, 1978) and F. Loux, *L'ogre et la dent*.

15. See in particular the collection edited by Daniel Roche (Montalba), reprinting popular literature.

16. Lise Andriès, 'Etude diachronique de la bibliothèque bleue et de son statut culturel aux 17e et 18e siècles', doctoral thesis (Paris, 1981). See also, Jean-Luc Marais, 'Littérature et culture "populaires" aux XVIIe et XVIIIe siècles. Réponses et questions', *Annales de Bretagne*, Mars 1980, no. 1, 65–106.

17. Jeanne Favret, *Deadly Words, Witchcraft in the Bocage*, trans. Catherine Cullen (Cambridge, 1980); Jeanne Favret and Josée Contreras, *Corps pour corps, Enquête sur la sorcellerie dans le Bocage* (Gallimard, 1981); 'Comment produire de l'energie avec deux jeux de cartes', *Bulletin d'ethno-médecine, 10* (1983), 3–57; 'L'embrayeur de violence. Quelques mécanismes thérapeutiques du désorcèlement' in J. Contreras, J. Favret-Saada, J. Hochmann, O. Mannoni and F. Roustang, *Le moi et l'autre* (Denoël, 1985).

18. Dan Sperber, *Le symbolisme en général* (Paris, Hermann, 1974).

19. See, Marc Auge and Claudine Herzlich, *Le sens du mal* (Paris, Maisons des Sciences de L'homme, 1984).

20. Mireille Laget and Claudine Luu, *D'aprés le livret de Dom Alexandre, Médecine et chirurgie des pauvres au 18e siècle* (Toulouse, Privat, 1984).

21. The work of Michel Leiris is important for an entire generation of French ethnologists, firstly on account of the intrinsic merit of his work, and secondly on account of his commitment to the form and to the literary corpus that he has led. The ethnologist's journey outside himself is at the same time also a journey inside himself, in which the imaginary plays an

important role.

22. Colette Petonnet, 'L'Observation flottante, l'exemple d'un cimetière parisien', *L'Homme, XXII* (1983), 37–47.

II

Medical History and Historical Demography

5

Methodological Problems in Modern Urban History Writing: Graphic Representations of Urban Mortality 1750–1850

Arthur E. Imhof

In European countries the exact registration of each death, indicating date of death, name, sex, age, trade or profession, cause of death, etc., was only generally introduced during the 16th, 17th or even 18th centuries. But since that time millions of people have died and large amounts of data have been preserved in the archives and offices of churches, cities or states, ready to be evaluated by historians, statisticians, demographers, genealogists, members of the medical profession, sociologists, economists and other interested people.

So as not to be drowned in this sea of figures, it is legitimate, even necessary, to limit one's scope; for instance, to 'Methodological problems in urban history: Demography and social stratification in the early phase of industrialisation (in Stockholm), 1750–1850'. However, the narrower the limitation, the greater the danger of myopic vision. Or to keep to the metaphor: one is inclined to regard one's little research island as *the* decisive mini-realm, as the only viable platform. I do not intend to disparage the value of special conferences and detailed studies that must exist. However, my present aim is to contribute to the relativisation of such a narrow vision and to draw attention to wider connections.

I will present my theme, 'Urban mortality 1750–1850' in the form of 12 'graphic mirror images' (Figures 5.1–5.12). My aim is to show how, from the figures we have, we can go on to consider the social factors that helped to form them. I have divided the 12 mirror images into six problem areas that represent deliberately diverse areas of my research, in order to show how in different ways one moves from demographic data to social history.

Arthur E. Imhof

Integration into a temporal and spatial mortality landscape (see Figures 5.1 and 5.2)

Figure 5.1 shows mortality in Berlin between 1721 and 1980. When this comparatively long period is considered as a whole, it is inevitable that other questions move to the foreground than would be the case with just the one hundred years between 1750 and 1850. In the former case, fundamental changes in the *structure* of mortality are the chief factor: from a phase of strongly oscillating but generally high mortality (until about 1810) through a quiet phase on a high level (until about 1870) and the demographic transition phase (until about 1930) to today's phase of equalised mortality on a low level. On the other hand, a myopic narrowing down to the years between 1750 and 1850 causes one more easily to ask about details of the earlier history of events, such as: what was it that brought about the peaks of 1758, 1763, 1771, 1808? (Answer: first the involvement of Berlin in the Seven Years' War 1756–1763, then the very bad harvests during the early 1770s and the French occupation during the Napoleonic War of 1806–1808). In this way questions that have recently become important for the history of mental attitudes such as the change in outlook regarding death and dying that occurred because of a gradual pacification and postponement of death during modern times do not get a chance of becoming relevant. They disappear from view because the observation period is too short. This type of periodisation makes for an 'old-fashioned' impression from the very beginning.

Figure 5.2 demonstrates the integration of 'urban mortality' into a spatial mortality landscape. Charted in the upper part is infant mortality within the German Empire during the years 1875–1877. A very clear structure emerges that is of a definite increase, on the one hand, from North to South and, on the other hand, from West to East. At the bottom, the results of seven micro-studies for the years 1780 to 1899 have been inserted into this landscape. All the cases, apart from Philippsburg, are concerned with rural areas. But equally, whether of town or of country, *each* study fits perfectly into its own landscape. From this one can conclude that the regional position of the place investigated is of prime importance for the incidence of mortality of its inhabitants; so that, for instance, this is of more significance than whether it is situated in town or countryside (in any case where it is a matter of small towns).

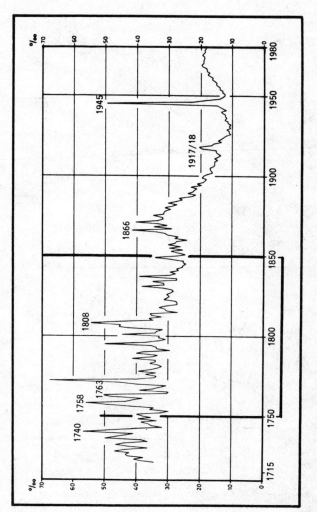

Figure 5.1: Mortality in Berlin 1721–1980. Data in promille (i.e. number of deaths per 1000 inhabitants).

Source: *Berliner Statistik, 31*, (1977), 8, frontispiece; also continuation to 1980 on the basis of data from the Statistiches Landesamt, Berlin.

Figure 5.2: Geography of infant mortality. Top: Infant mortality within the confines of the German Empire 1875–1877. Bottom: Micro-studies fitted into their geographical unit. No matter whether town (like Philippsburg) or country (all others), all of them fit perfectly into their landscape. It must not be forgotten, however, that Philippsburg, at the time, had a maximum of 2600 inhabitants.

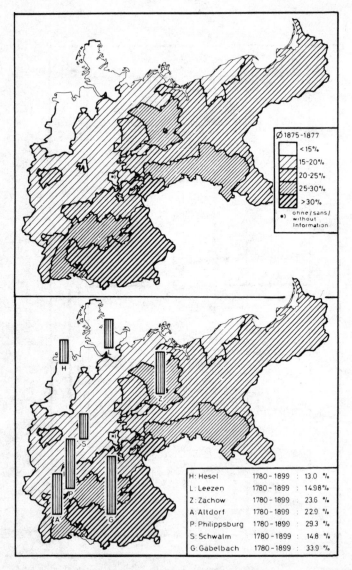

H: Hesel	1780 – 1899	:	13.0 %
L: Leezen	1780 – 1899	:	14.98%
Z: Zachow	1780 – 1899	:	23.6 %
A: Altdorf	1780 – 1899	:	22.9 %
P: Philippsburg	1780 – 1899	:	29.3 %
S: Schwalm	1780 – 1899	:	14.8 %
G: Gabelbach	1780 – 1899	:	33.9 %

Source: *Zeitschrift für Bevölkerungswissenschaft*, 7 (1981), 363.

Interaction between town and country (Figures 5.3–5.5)

Town and countryside complemented each other at all times, not only sharing the workload but also with regard to population. For both of them, however, a phase of intensified urbanisation and industrialisation had a series of serious consequences during the 18th and 19th centuries.

In Figure 5.3 we see on the right hand the development of the population of Nedertoneå at the end of the Bottnic gulf at the frontier between Sweden and Finland between 1820 and 1880. This parish, which is spread over a large area, originally consisted of a number of larger and smaller rural settlements. After the lost war against Russia and the realignment of the frontier back to the river Torne at the peace treaty of Fredrikshamn in 1809, one of them, the bridgehead Haparanda, received successive civil rights during the 1830s and 1840s and was systematically extended to become a proper frontier fortress. From then on a distinction was made between an urban and a rural parish. Not only did Haparanda increase rapidly from that time onwards, being strongly favoured by the State (1850, 472 inhabitants; 1880, 1060), but it became inundated with a set of Swedish-speaking non-indigenous officials, military persons and tradesmen who, from the point of view of cultural geography, were oriented in a different direction from the original population surrounding them, which was traditionally rooted in agriculture and spoke Finnish. Villages like Vuono, Nikkala, Mattila and Vojakala, situated near the town of Haparanda and accessible to traffic, however, were drawn more and more into the sphere of influence exerted by the market of the fast expanding city centre. On the one hand, they became suppliers of agricultural products such as milk, meat, grain and vegetables needed in Haparanda in ever larger quantities; on the other hand, they succumbed increasingly to the efforts towards acculturation made by the city, for instance, the massive campaign by doctors and midwives for the care of nursing mothers and their babies. Yet the more mothers went over to the suckling of their own babies, following the example of urban Swedish women, the more they were hit by the consequences of lactation amenorrhoea. In the left half of Figure 5.3 it can be easily recognised that, in this way, the traditional seasonal rhythm of births, which had been heretofore beneficial to babies and mothers, became disturbed and postponed to the summertime, which was unfavourable for mothers and babies (especially so in 1845–1869).

Arthur E. Imhof

Figure 5.3: The parish of Nedertorneå on the frontier between Sweden and Finland at the end of the Bottnic Gulf 1820–1894. Originally this extensive parish consisted of a series of larger and smaller villages. When one of them, Haparanda at the border river Torne, obtained successive civic rights during the 1830s, a distinction was made, after this, between an urban and a rural parish of Nedertorneå. Left: Distribution of births, respectively conceptions calculated for nine months earlier, in the rural parish of Nedertorneå during the periods of 1820–1844, 1845–1869 and 1870–1894. Standardised calculation for 1200 cases per period and a uniform length of months of 30 days. Starting with the second period it becomes clear how the traditional rhythm of conceptions and births was moved on by several months because of the increasing number of mothers breastfeeding their babies and the lactation amenorrhoea connected with this. Right: Development of the population in the rural (= L for land) and the urban (= H for Haparanda town) parishes of Nedertorneå in 1820, 1850 and 1880. The two largest villages of the rural area were Vuono and Nikkala. Amongst the medium ones were Säivits, Mattila, Neder-land Över-Vojakala, amongst the small ones were Leipijärvi, Nartijärvi and Pitkäjärvi. Whereas the large and medium villages were situated along the main road leading to Haparanda Town and, therefore, were drawn more quickly into the sphere of market relations with it, the small villages were situated apart on by-roads.

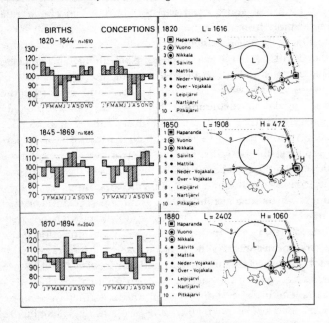

Source: Anders Brändström, *De kärlekslösa mödrarna, Spädbarnsdödligheten i Sverige under 1800–talet med särskild hänsyn till Nedertorneå församling* (Stockholm, Almqvist & Wiksell, 1984), table 7, figure 8 and supplement IID. In the right-hand compartments of the graphic the radius of each circle, not its surface, is proportional to the size of the population in the rural, or the city parish, respectively.

Nevertheless, because of the greater number of breastfeeding mothers the infant mortality in the countryside eventually was reduced from over 300 per thousand during 1845–1869 to under 250 during 1870–1895 (cf. Figure 5.4 left). But what was the gain? More babies survived their first year of life, but more died more frequently afterwards as infants, after having been weaned. Certainly, it can be seen clearly from the right-hand-side of the illustration that during the same observation period the mortality of children between one and five years old (months of life 13–60) increased considerably. The ratio in the city of Haparanda had been similar to this all the time, that is, there was a lower infant mortality than in the rural community because suckling by the mothers was generally practised. Conversely, the mortality of small children was substantially higher than in the countryside. Moreover, from the same illustration it can be seen that infant mortality in Haparanda city between 1845–1869 and 1870–1895 rose remarkably and finally reached nearly the same level as that in the rural areas. This deterioration did not occur because mothers stopped breastfeeding their babies but because the city was growing too rapidly. The hygienic conditions deteriorated (the provision of drinking water and sewage drains) to such an extent that a number of infectious diseases claimed more and more victims, including babies.[1]

Figure 5.5. shows some of the ambivalent positive-negative consequences of symbioses of the culture, economy and population of town and countryside. Admittedly the endogenous mortality (during the first month of life) was at all times lower in the city because of the more favourable perinatal conditions (such as better-trained midwives, specialist obstetricians and lying-in hospitals) than in the rural areas, and those progressive circumstances also benefited in the end, after some delay, the countryside, so that there, too, endogenous neonatal mortality gradually receded (cf. Figure 5.5). But, on the other hand, we also notice during the same observation period an increase in infant mortality. While this increase in the rapidly growing towns, as attested now for Haparanda, goes back to the negative consequences of comparative over-population, it can be explained for the rural areas rather by the overworking of women and mothers in the agricultural concerns that had become more and more included in the marketing sphere of the towns. For instance, mothers had no time to breast feed their babies but instead of keeping fresh cows' milk for them to drink, they sold it down to the last drop at lucrative prices to the insatiable towns.[2]

Arthur E. Imhof

Figure 5.4: The mortality of infants and small children in the rural and in the urban parish of Nedertorneå during the first five years of life. Top: 1845–1869 (in Haparanda town only 1855–1859). Bottom: 1870–1895 (in Haparanda town only 1885–1889). The two columns on the left always denote neonatal mortality per 1000 live births during months 0–12, the two columns on the right, months 13–60. Note the different scales. While neonatal mortality during the first period was considerably higher in the rural areas than in the town, and the opposite ratio was true for infant mortality, during the second period neonatal mortality had indeed decreased but now far more infants died during the months directly after: a result of increasing rural suckling during the first year of life.

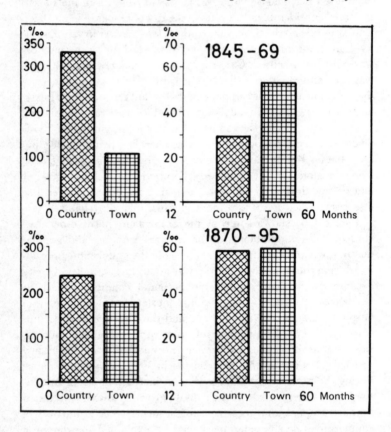

Source: Anders Brändström, *De kärlekslösa mödrarna. Spädbarnsdödligheten i Sverige under 1800-talet med särskild hänsyn till Nedertorneå församling* (Stockholm, Almqvist & Wiksell, 1984), Figure 26 and Table 16.

Figure 5.5: Development of infant mortality as well as mortality according to chiefly endogenous causes (hatched area in circle, deaths during first month of life), and exogenous causes (bar, months 2–12) during the period of 1780–1899. Left: In the city of Philippsburg. Right: In the four farming villages Altdorf, Gabelbach, Hesel and Zachow.

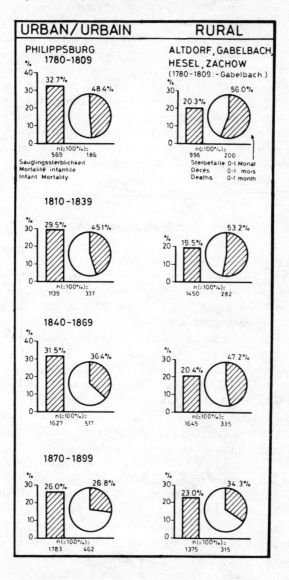

We should also consider whether the towns definitely served as reservoirs for the surplus population from the rural areas and thus relieved pressure in a positive manner; or whether the towns were capable of preserving or increasing their number of inhabitants only in this way, as were under constant threat of being depopulated due to the higher mortality of urban as opposed to country areas. Conversely, however, it was only the young people, and often the best and most active, who left the rural areas. This resulted, as is well known, in a city-oriented population structure (in a similar way nowadays through the 'guest workers', in countries allowing temporary immigration). Continuous bloodletting on the one hand, a new lease of life through new blood on the other, were the result. Admittedly, only the city profited from this migration during which an innovative potential of supernumerary young men and women flowed into it while these people during 'the best years of their lives' were absent from the countryside.[3]

'Specific' mortalities (Figures 5.6 and 5.7)

For quite some time 'social inequality when faced with disease, old age, dying and death' has been one of the favourite subjects among economic and social historians and historian-demographers.[4] But, with the aid of Figure 5.6, I am not going to make the obvious connections once again. What I want to do is to make one question the central one, that is, the effect of such circumstances as prevailed then on the different social strata. Thus I do not mean to demonstrate the fact or to explain why population class IV in Halle on the Saale 1855–1875 suffered from a rate of still-births and mortality of infants and small children twice as high as that for the highest class (officials, doctors, lawyers, wholesale merchants), or why deaths from infections and other acute diseases were much more frequent in the former class than with the latter. I want rather to suggest that the people from stratum I, whether we like it or not, have much more in common with us than those of stratum IV. The reason for this is not because we probably belong to a class more closely related to them, but because of a profile regarding age of death and a spectrum of causes of death much more similar to ours than is the case with the lower stratum. At that time developments started in the upper stratum that concerns us *all* today. Some of these were the rise in the ratio of old people to the total population, the small number of children, death from heart and circulatory disease, death from 'decrepitude' and as a consequence: an increase in the problems and conflicts of the generations, with parents or bosses at work or in the professions and those in control of politics, the economy, society and power living longer; a longer waiting period for an inheritance — which increasingly skipped a whole generation — psychological problems of couples whose children had grown up and who spent an ever longer time together once the family had grown up, problems of longer widowhoods at the end of life, etc.

The whole complex of problems seems nowadays very familiar to us all. But at the time it was, to a large extent, exclusively a problem of the upper social stratum. At least against this background the circumstances at the time amongst the less privileged strata of the population were not *merely* disadvantageous to the young people.

Another subject frequently dealt with in recent times on the part of historical demographers and medical historians concerned with specific mortalities is the mortality of mothers. Admittedly, these studies hardly ever referred exclusively to the towns.[5] Recent comparative studies on town and countryside showed that during the period of 1780–1899 generally, that is, not only in the towns or only in the countryside, there was a preponderance of mortality among women of childbearing age. In these population surveys the husbands were used always as controls. From Figure 5.7, which shows the result for the city of Philippsburg, it becomes clear that the conjecture usually suggested at first, namely that the cause for this was the high mortality of mothers is *not* true. Even when the deaths during or after childbed are left out of consideration (marked in the illustration by black domes), there still remains a preponderance of the mortality amongst these women. My explanation of this is that married women of childbearing age in town and country had to bear simultaneously a threefold burden that only by a *convergence* led to this preponderance in mortality: first, a heavy or even more intensified workload in the household, in the stable, on the farm, in the fields, in the factory; secondly, they were being heavily burdened with a mother's responsibilities due to a comparatively high birthrate persisting as before; and thirdly, a new burden was laid upon them by the outside world — they become the central personality in the family in the context of campaigns of hygienisation, enlightenment and education on the part of the State.[6] In this area investigations of specific social strata in expanding, industrialised cities would be very desirable because they could furnish valuable further results.

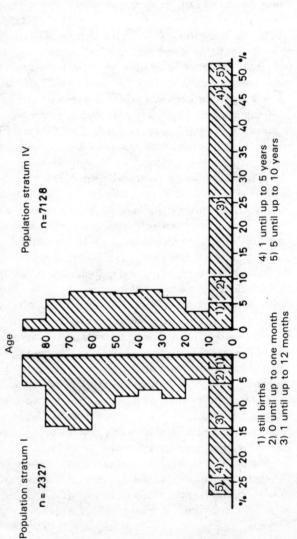

Figure 5.6: Social inequality with reference to dying and death in the city of Halle on the Saale, 1855–1875. Top: Distribution of deaths in two different social strata according to their age at death. Data in per cent (100 per cent = all deaths in the relevant stratum). Bottom: Distribution of deaths in two different social strata according to their cause of death. Data in per cent (100 per cent = all deaths in the relevant stratum). In each case left: Population stratum I: Senior officials, physicians, lawyers, clergymen, wholesale merchants. In each case on the right: Population stratum IV: Service personnel, manual and factory workers, untrained employees.

Spectrum of causes of death

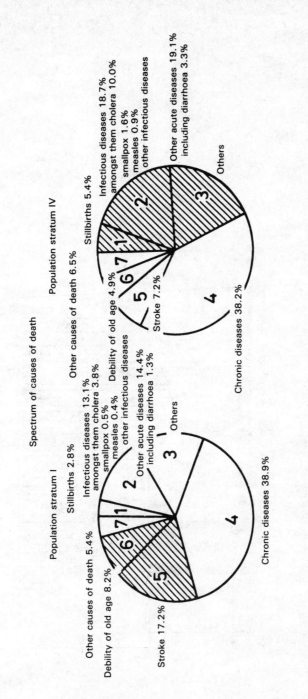

Population stratum I

Other causes of death 5.4%
Stillbirths 2.8%
Infectious diseases 13.1%
amongst them cholera 3.8%
smallpox 0.5%
measles 0.4%
other infectious diseases
Debility of old age 8.2%
Other acute diseases 14.4%
including diarrhoea 1.3%
Others
Stroke 17.2%
Chronic diseases 38.9%

Population stratum IV

Stillbirths 5.4%
Other causes of death 6.5%
Infectious diseases 18.7%
amongst them cholera 10.0%
smallpox 1.6%
measles 0.9%
other infectious diseases
Other acute diseases 19.1%
including diarrhoea 3.3%
Debility of old age 4.9%
Others
Stroke 7.2%
Chronic diseases 38.2%

Source: J. Conrad: *Beitrag zur Untersuchung des Einflusses von Lebensstellung und Beruf auf die Mortalitätsverhältnisse, auf Grund des statistischen Materials* at Halle on the Saale 1855–74 (Jena, 1877), 59–60, 152.

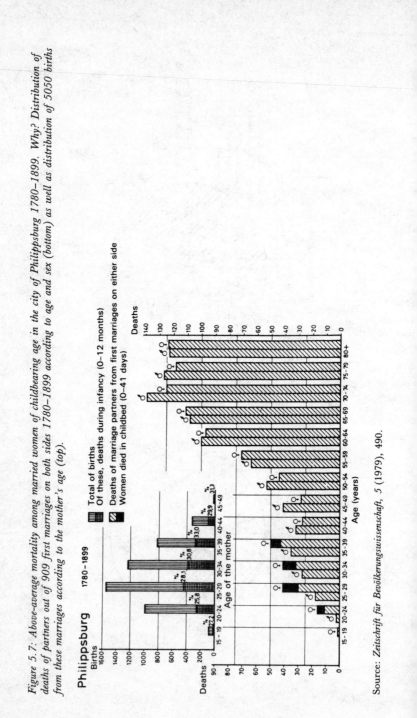

Figure 5.7: Above-average mortality among married women of childbearing age in the city of Philippsburg 1780–1899. Why? Distribution of deaths of partners out of 909 first marriages on both sides 1780–1899 according to age and sex (bottom) as well as distribution of 5050 births from these marriages according to the mother's age (top).

40,000 deaths in the Berlin parish of Dorotheenstadt 1715–1875: What questions?

One of our data banks in Berlin contains information relating to around 40,000 deaths in the Berlin parish of Dorotheenstadt between 1715 and 1875. Of course, it is no problem for the computer to produce on command all possible print-outs and to carry out any calculations asked for. But at the end nothing would come out except reams and reams of computer paper — resulting in a lot of resigned frustration. As we know, the calculating machine does not offer enclosures with meaningful explanations. So it is still up to the researcher, when undertaking any large-scale programming, to formulate questions guided by theory and to think over carefully what questions he wants answered. Then, indeed, the computer becomes an indispensable aid and an extremely helpful partner.

First of all, it can pay to plot a chart with the proportional distribution of all deaths per hundred within the most important age groups during the recorded 160 years. We then establish that, during this period, evidently no radical changes took place with regard to age groups. Certain instructive tendencies, however, are unmistakable, as, for instance, the rising rate of still-births in the course of the 19th century or the increasing infant mortality and simultaneous decreasing mortality. Finally there is a clear indication that the average population of Berlin became increasingly older. The number of deaths among the adult, the elderly and those of advanced old age was rising considerably.

The sudden break shortly after 1800 when vaccination against smallpox had become therapeutically effective should not be overlooked and neither should the disturbing rebound of baby mortality to its original rate after hardly a generation. Although the vaccinated babies no longer died of smallpox, stomach and intestinal complaints and those of the respiratory organs took its place more or less immediately in the panorama of causes of death. Was this a good exchange? The historian is beginning to speculate!

But it was a very concrete matter for the mothers of the time. Suddenly, because of a fundamentally changed pathological situation, a considerably greater importance was given to suckling. Gastro-intestinal impairments to health correlated incomparably more frequently with neglected lactation than with the ravages of smallpox.

But the same background may elicit quite a different question, for instance, when looking at the data relating to the deaths from smallpox and the waves of cholera since the 1830s. In both cases it was a matter of infectious diseases causing epidemics that appeared according to periodic rhythms. But the great difference between them was the fact that smallpox decimated a marginal age group of little social consequence (that is, babies and infants), while cholera afflicted *all* age groups, including those most important for the functioning of society, those in 'the best years of their lives' and in positions of power. Although cholera demanded numerically fewer victims it was an incomparably greater social menace. Those empowered to use all kinds of measures acted with corresponding swiftness and effectiveness. While smallpox had been allowed for centuries to be rampant practically unchecked, cholera was brought under control within a few generations. Threats posed by fatal diseases to the whole of society have at all times been less tolerated than those specific to marginal age groups, be they, as then, concentrated within the youngest age group or, as today, within the older and oldest age groups.

Causes of death: What has changed? (Figures 5.8–5.11)

Practically all of our roughly 40,000 death entries also contained indications on the cause of death; within the European framework, especially for the first half of the century, this is something of a rarity. From a computer print-out on the frequency distribution per year of the roughly 3,000 entries for causes of death, we find, as expected, great changes during this span of more than one and a half centuries. The disappearance of smallpox and the ensuing boom in gastro-intestinal complaints amongst babies and infants and the appearance of cholera, a new epidemic disease imported from Asia, has already been mentioned. Yet in the following pages I shall not go into details of biological changes of this kind, however important for medical history, but rather point to even profounder transformations that initially produce great difficulties for our understanding of the dynamics of the range of causes of death.[7]

Let us look at Figure 5.8, in which the computer has listed the 3,164 deaths caused by 'feverish complaints' for every five years. Up to the end of the 18th century the foreground was taken unequivocally by 'acute fever' (658 cases), simply 'fever' (448) or 'hectic fever' (151). Around 1800 a notable change occurred. Then just as unequivocally 'scarlet fever' (324 cases) or 'nerve

Figure 5.8: Distribution of deaths from the most important feverish complaints (designation of causes of death containing the word stem 'fever') in the Berlin parish of Dorotheenstadt according to their emergence in time per quinquennium 1715–1875. Data in absolute figures.

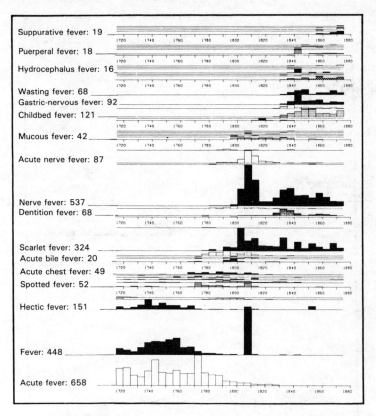

Source: Data bank based on the death registers of the parish of Dorotheenstadt; Evangelical Central Archive, Berlin (West). Plotted computer graphic.

fever' (537) as well as a whole series of special forms of fever such as 'mucous fever' (42), 'gastric-nervous fever' (92) or 'hydrocephalus fever' (16) moved to the central position. On the other hand, the disease names that before had been frequently used disappeared completely, not because the older forms of fever did not exist any longer, but because the nomenclature of causes of death had become different. Causes of death are labels that

Figure 5.9: Distribution of deaths from liver complaints (designations of causes of death containing the word stem 'liver' or 'hepat') in the Berlin parish of Dorotheenstadt according to their emergence in time per quinquennium 1715–1875. Data in absolute figures.

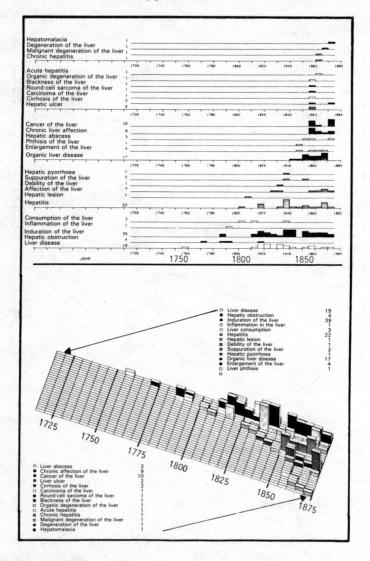

Source: Data bank based on the death registers of the parish of Dorotheenstadt; Evangelical Central Archive, Berlin (West). Plotted computer graphic.

Figure 5.10: Distribution of deaths from 'teething' (designations of causes of death containing the word stems 'teeth' or 'dent') in the Berlin parish of Dorotheenstadt 1715–1875. Data in absolute figures. Top: According to their emergence in time per quinquennium. Bottom: Number of cases each year (marked as black columns).

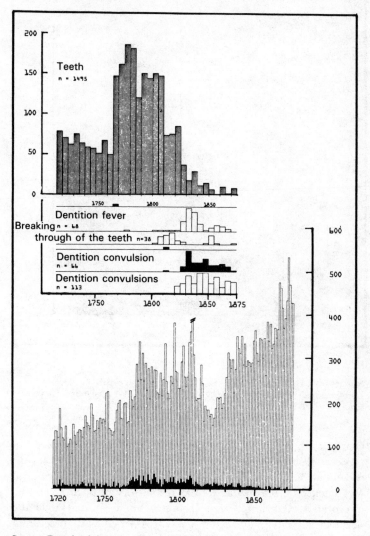

Source: Data bank based on the death registers of the parish of Dorotheenstadt; Evangelical Central Archive, Berlin (West). Plotted computer graphic.

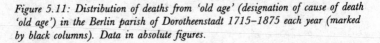

Figure 5.11: Distribution of deaths from 'old age' (designation of cause of death 'old age') in the Berlin parish of Dorotheenstadt 1715–1875 each year (marked by black columns). Data in absolute figures.

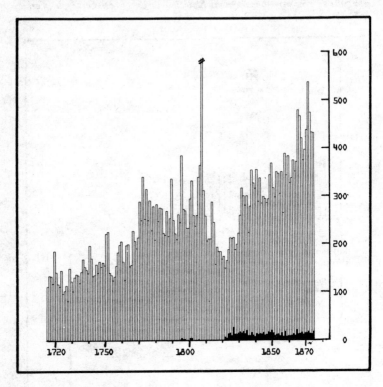

Source: Data bank based on the death registers of the parish of Dorotheenstadt; Evangelical Central Archive, Berlin (West). Plotted computer graphic.

change with the viewpoint of the labeller. Each terminology of causes of death, including our own, is attached to a system. It can, therefore, only be understood within a larger context of cultural and intellectual history as well as the history of science, and be interpreted accordingly. For instance, up to around 1800 the nosological system of the day was concerned with describing symptoms, and people died of striking symptoms easily recognisable by any lay person. The 'acute fever' was the decisive criterion, not this or that infectious disease underlying it. When, with increasing medical knowledge, the aetiological system replaced the observation of symptoms with the investigation of causes, the decisive criterion was no longer the symptom, that is, no longer the feverish condition, but the infectious disease at the bottom of it, for instance, scarlet fever.

As historians we should always ask questions about the implications of such changes and we must not forget that with the transformation of the 'physician's viewpoint' from that of the symptoms of disease to that of the causes of disease a change began in the doctor-patient relationship, the results of which can be felt even today. There was a move away from a sick *person* suffering from symptoms to the dysfunction of particular organs or cells. The doctor began to penetrate deeper and deeper under the patient's skin, and was increasingly losing sight of the whole personality.

In Figure 5.9 I want to show once again in graphic form how this process of gradual splitting-up and parcelling out progresses. The old comprehensive terms for the various kinds of fever suffered by the sick are resolved more and more into scientific details centering on organs, until, in the end, people are being said to have died of 'nervous bile fever', of 'rheumatic nervous fever', of 'abdominal nerve fever', and of 'catarrhal fever' and so on. With the 'liver'-centred causes of death (in Figure 5.9) the development described is even more obvious. They can, of course, only occur after the liver has been 'discovered' as an organ no longer functioning properly. At first it was a matter of rather general terminology: 'liver disease' (19 cases), but after 1800 here, too, occurred a rapid differentiation extending further and further right up to one case each of 'carcinoma of the liver', 'round cell sarcoma of the liver', 'blackening of the liver', and 'organic degeneration of the liver' — none of these being visible from the outside.

How is it that hundreds of babies and infants up to around 1800 were dying of 'teeth' (1495 cases, see Figure 5.10)? This can now easily be understood. The painful breaking through of the first milk teeth could not be overlooked by those around the baby because of the baby's bawling and whimpering. If babies happened to die during that period they obviously died of this perceptible symptom, the 'teeth'. Here, too, the appellation gradually disappears after 1800. At the lower margin of the graph we see, however, a further development that I take up again in Figure 5.11. Just as we have been talking of a 'change in the physician's viewpoint' and of the 'discovery' of diseased inner organs as the cause of death, we can talk here of a 'change in the social view-point' and the discovery of the two marginal age groups, that is, 'infancy' and 'old age'. It is true, that there were no purely numerical reasons for this to have happened during the period investigated. There was no particular moment when there was a sudden increase or decrease in the number of deaths of either babies and infants or old people. And yet, since the 1820s, the deaths of 'old age' increase (Figure 5.11 at the bottom) and the deaths of 'teeth', at times nearly identical with infant mortality altogether, decrease considerably, and in the end they nearly disappear totally. Their place was taken more and more by very specific children's diseases. The 'attention' of parents, physicians and society focused increasingly on these hitherto neglected age groups. Here, too, the change in the range of causes of death is explicable less in terms of the history of biology than this history of mental attitudes and culture.

Disease — dying — death in the context of the cosmic order and metaphysics (Figure 5.12)

In all the preceding sections I have repeatedly tried to fit each special type of mortality problem into a larger context: micro-regional studies into a mortality landscape, short-term period investigations into longer stretches of time, the study of towns into their root conditions in the countryside, changing ranges of death into the framework not only of the history of biology and medicine, but also of processes belonging to the history of society, of attitudes and of culture.

With the last figure I should like to draw attention to a further overall context that we have increasingly lost sight of, but which has been of great importance to the majority of our ancestors until recently, that is the fact that the ideas on disease — dying — death used to form part of a metaphysical cosmic mental pattern. This can be demonstrated by looking more closely at the 3,164 deaths from 'feverish complaints' that had occurred in 1715–1875 in the Berlin parish of Dorotheenstadt, but this time according to age at death. It appears that throughout the whole period people of all ages were affected continually by fever. This was, therefore, a matter of everyday relevance in contrast to the children's disease of smallpox or the cholera epidemics that occurred only sporadically. This kind of health risk was present always and

Figure 5.12: Schematic representation of successive occidental ideas about life and its duration: in Homeric-Old Testament times, during about 2000 years of the New Testament-metaphysical epoch, as well as the post-metaphysical period of today.

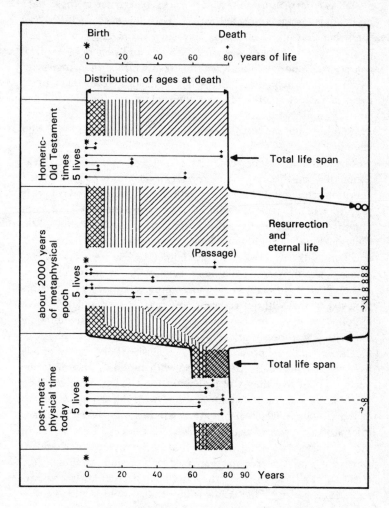

Sources and inspirations: Walter Schulz, 'Wandlungen der Einstellung zum Tode', in Johannes Schwartländer (ed.) *Der Mensch und sein Tod*, Göttingen, Vandenhoeck & Ruprecht, 1976), 94–107; Joachim Whaley (ed.) *Mirrors of mortality. Studies in the social history of death* (London, Europa Publications, 1981); Karl Stüber, *Commendatio animae. Sterben im Mittelalter* (Bern, Herbert Lang, 1976); Bernard Guillemain *et al.* (ed.), *La mort au moyen âge* (Strasbourg, Librairie Istra, 1977); Roger Chartier *et al.*, *La mort aujourd'hui* (Marseille, Éditions Rivages, 1982).

everywhere. It was part of the scheme of things. One had just got used to it, just as one had got used to the coldness of winter or the darkness of the night. Like the winter coldness and nightly darkness it formed a natural part of the experience of those days and the viewpoint connected with it. This, however, included also the belief that a loss of health was a sign from Heaven to mend one's ways while there was time. Prayers and penances were, of course, the more suitable reactions to this rather than treatment by orthodox medicine and medicaments or paramedical practices.[8] Diseases, therefore, had their place in this view of the world, just as dying and death, which, at that time, did not signify the end but only the passing over from existence in this life to that beyond it.

The schematic representation of successive occidental ideas about 'life' and its duration expresses even more poignantly the enormous changes that occurred in the course of hundreds of years (Figure 5.12). During the time of Homer and the Old Testament our ancestors seem to have been very conscious of their mortality. Only during the roughly two thousand years of the 'metaphysical' epoch did Christian beliefs as proclaimed by the New Testament, develop about resurrection and eternal life in heavenly bliss. Although it is difficult to say how many amongst our ancestors believed in this without reservations, it is likely that four of five hypothetical lives were provided with the sign for infinity and only one with a question mark. Nowadays, in the post-metaphysical, secularised age, the proportion is the opposite. For four out of five lives dying and death are identical with the end, and only one person out of five may still believe in the Christian eternal life.

As studies on mortality always deal with the dying and death of individuals it seems also appropriate to probe every time into their world view and beliefs in order to understand what death means to them. Is it not possible that in the metaphysical epoch, which for many people has vanished only a short time ago, the duration of a lifespan on earth would have been of far less importance than for us? This is not to say that people would not also have felt attached to earthly life and have been afraid of dying and death.[9] The comparative 'less' is meant in relation to us for whom, after the loss of belief in eternal life, the earthly phase of life has become identical with life as such.

Against this background it is hardly adequate to direct our investigations on mortality, for instance, as here, for the period 1750–1850, solely towards finding out which groups, strata, classes, parts of the population used to have shorter or longer lives, where the mortality of infants, children and adults was lowest or highest or where it experienced the greatest reduction. Such questions are posed from *our, today's* point of view, not from the perspectives of that time and its people. Being historians, we really ought to endeavour to do a little more justice to our ancestors by trying to see *their* world with *their* eyes and to judge it by their own standards.

Afterword

As I had the honour to open the Cambridge Conference on Problems and Methods in the History of Medicine with my presentation, I used this extraordinary position pedagogically in two ways: first by merely presenting an original twenty — hopefully attractive and 'speaking' (expressive) — figures showing the main conclusions I have come to in my research during the past decade, I introduced and involved the participants more and more deeply in the general conference topic and I tried to stimulate as many of them as possible to give reactions and comments in a very broad and all-embracing opening discussion. And second — since the participants had come from many different disciplines and research fields as well as from different countries — I tried to learn as much as possible from their eminent capacities for my future research.

Let us first take a look at the result of this approach, as one of the participants after the Conference put it:

> The central aim of the meeting was to examine methodological problems now facing historians of medicine in the light of recent developments in historiography, in particular the impact of quantitative analysis and computer technology. The discussion inevitably became focused on a comparison of the traditional scholarship of qualitative research into historical 'events', with high technology, statistical explanations of changing 'trends' in historical structures. In this context, the opening session presented by Arthur Imhof set out clearly the terms of the subsequent debate. His aim was to demonstrate the necessity of an interdisciplinary approach to studies such as his own current work on the historical demography of family reconstitution. Imhof

claimed that a complex analysis of statistical trends in population changes described the appearance of historical relations but did not provide an understanding of them. For the latter he sought documentation from manuscript and archival texts, paintings, sculptures and artefacts; and, when possible for the modern period, oral accounts of the past from individuals who experienced it. During the exchange which followed Imhof's presentation, it became clear that he believed the dialectic of historiography to be inherently linked to the dialectic of historical relations themselves. Investigation of the past, for Imhof, revealed the underlying realities of the present. The methodological discourse which he considered to be dominated by his sources was matched by discourses between what has been, what is and what ought to be the structure of our social organisations, for example in the social relations of health and disease.[10]

But now, *after* the presentation of the paper, *after* the discussions are over, after the conference altogether, and thus no longer trying to influence the participants from the very beginning, I may be allowed to add some concluding remarks, merely as food for thought for the reader. I could not express my aim better than by quoting Ashish Bose, President of the Indian Association for the Study of Population, when he addressed the Tenth Annual Conference of his Society in Bangalore in May 1985:

I welcome the recent developments in India and abroad to abandon Demography in favour of Population Studies or Population Sciences. However, things do not improve merely by changing the nomenclature. The orientation, quality and scope must also change to make it a meaningful science relevant to planning and policy making. My exhortation to my fellow demographers at this stage would be: 'Look beyond the decimal points.' Of course, one must *begin* by looking at the decimal points but one should not get stuck for ever in the decimal point,'

and ending with:

We should abandon the number game and move from population to people.[11]

The basic method in historical demography, i.e. the family reconstitution method, makes it easy to follow this exhortation. Before we reconstitute the families of the 16th, 17th, 18th, 19th or 20th centuries on the basis of entries in dozens of registers of baptisms, marriages and deaths, and compile them into data banks and feed the results into the computer, we look at every individual person in the parish registers. We know his or her name, the birth, marriage and death date, his or her parents, partners and children, we know where and how long he or she has lived, and many other things. That is, we know thousands of *individual lives* as they actually happened at a given time. In the same way we know *individual families*. As I see it we should remain much longer with these individual lives and individual families and should kindle our imagination with this reconstructed material and be inspired by it. *A population, after all, is always individual persons.* Or, to quote Pierre Goubert, a masterly historian of French everyday peasant life, from whom I have learned an immense amount with regard to 'Historical Demography beyond Decimal Points':

> To dip deeply, up to the point of being pleasantly submerged, into the landscapes, the stones, the books, the oral tradition of an old society before it goes to pieces. To attack it from all sides with all the means at one's disposal, to be at home in it as if on one's own ground and to feel its life pulsating through all its pores. Slowly to reconstruct that life and, what is more, not only that of the 'great ones': that is the historian's task. Quite simply a recreation, within knowable limits, which demands, above all, courage, humility and conscientiousness in order to be valid, and, if possible, attentive sympathy and an ounce of finesse.[12]

Yet, whatever amount of empathy we develop during our years as historical demographers and historians of everyday history, with our thus by no means nameless ancestors, we shall never go so far as to become nostalgic. Because who would want to exchange our conditions of life with their's, remembering that, at that time, one's very existence was being constantly physically endangered? It is the historian of people's mentality above all who will never forget the line from the All-Saints' Litany, which encompasses those calamities so concisely and precisely: 'From pestilence, hunger and war preserve us, O Lord!'

Let us try to do one thing against this extended background:

127

to go again into the details of the first and the last diagrams (Figures 5.1 and 5.12). Regarding Figure 5.1, 'pure' historical demographers as well as general historians have usually over-looked or considered too little that the annual rates of mortality had ebbed considerably, e.g. in Berlin during the first half of the 19th century, even before they decreased within the framework of the demographic transition, from the early high figures down to today's level. We shall surely have to explain in detail and, no doubt, be able to do so with the help of historians of medicine and of economics, what were the reasons for this: for instance, the absence of plague and smallpox, the improvement of the infra-structure whereby the state provided better supply possibilities when there was a bad harvest, etc.

But if we have gone, as Goubert has taught us above, beyond statistics and have concentrated on the then everyday world of our ancestors, while intensively communicating with historians of folklore or with historians of religious attitudes, very different ideas will strike us on comtemplating this diagram. For many generations it was one of the recurring experiences of our ancestors that, at more or less short intervals, there appeared 'black peaks' in the population development, that is, that during this or that year always far more people died than were born. As most of our farming ancestors were living in 'deserts as far as accessibility of physicians was concerned' and were helplessly confronted with many infectious diseases leading to epidemics, they took refuge in this or that particular Saint provided by popular religion. Even today most of us know, at least from hear-say, Saint Sebastian or Saint Rochus as the 'Plague Saints'. Now my question is: what happened to those Saints when the plague disappeared? Did they thereby lose their right to exist? Without wishing to argue monocausally, it is at least worth considering whether this development did not form one of the contributory factors that lessened the influence of Christianity, and began, or spread more quickly, the secularisation of our outlook? The heavens began to be 'depopulated'.

From here we may continue immediately by looking at Figure 5.12. In the lower half of the figure there is a variation of what we have seen already in the first figure. For many centuries the ages at death encompassed a wide range and, therefore, the length of the total life-span differed considerably. Admittedly, it is likely that many people at the time believed, as they were told by the Christian Church through its teaching of the New Testament, in a resurrection of the flesh and an eternal life. Meanwhile our earthly life spans have now become largely standardised and reached a fairly equal length, but, at the same time, many amongst us have lost the belief in eternity. We find ourselves in something of a predicament because most of us still know, by dint of a long collective memory, just what we have forfeited in recent times.

To this must be added the point that clearly the standardising of our life-spans on earth has not yet been completed. There are still many people who die an 'untimely death'. While our physiological life expectation, that is, the average maximal life-span of the human species, should come to about 85 years, the actually lived life-span of the most of our fellow-men amounts to 10 or 15 years less. This goes back to the fact that, though the earlier infectious and parasitic causes of death have been eliminated, they have been replaced by chronic ailments. Therefore death, for many of us, no longer occurs swiftly, but slowly and painfully. In this regard we find ourselves in a nasty predicament.

In spite of this, the historian has no reason to see the future in a pessimistic light. It is true that he must be extremely careful each time he extrapolates from historical data. Things can turn out very differently from what had been predicted. But if the developments of the last decades or even centuries continue as before in the near future, ecological and physiological expectations of life could, on the whole, coincide. What that means is that more and more people would actually live out their life span of about 85 years. This state of affairs would be brought about if the thresholds of the onset of symptoms for today's chief causes of death, that is, above all, cardiovascular diseases and cancer, could be raised, to become apparent at an age that would have reached the limits of the life-span. Then we would have again, as during the time of the infectious diseases of our ancestors that killed swiftly, a swift, 'kind' death but — unlike them — at the end of a long and healthy life, practically down to the last breath. We would not then have to fear either an infinitely dragged out, painful inability to die or dependencies of all kinds at an advanced age.

Question after question emerges here, and all of them may very soon become relevant to the individual (because every one of us is going to die some time — the question is how?), to families, to society, to the state. Therefore, giving some thought to the issues today rather than tomorrow is worthwhile. Of course, it is not my job as a historian to give a competent answer to all problems. My task is to show where we stand today, to indicate the development of the last three or four hundred years, that is, to make diagnoses and not prognoses.

But there are questions about the future that we should consider. For instance, shall we become, when the physical pressure of 'pestilence, hunger and war' has been removed, a 'people of lone wolves'? Lone wolves are, in principle, not fertile. Will, therefore, a people that, for the first time in history, has reached this stage, that is, where, for the first time, ecological and physiological life expectations coincide, have passed its zenith and be sentenced to 'die out'? Is man not a 'social being' at all but was only forced into forming communities because of historically adverse circumstances?

And what about the 'lost eternity'? Could it not be that this 'eternity' was 'invented' not so much for the sake of the survivors but for that of the many non-survivors, that is, all those who, in the past, have died 'too early' and for whom there had to be somewhere some kind of compensation so that justice should prevail. But if all fellow-men could live, in a standardised way, equally long to the age of about 85, we should, of course, no longer need this 'eternity for the others'. And what about ourselves? If we had a long, healthy life guaranteed down to the last breath, if we could get here on earth everything desirable, what should we need an eternity for?

As I said before: it may not happen this way. But neither is it impossible if we consider the developments during the last few centuries; on the contrary, it is quite likely.[13] Therefore we have neither occasion to long, with inappropriate nostalgia, for the 'good old times' which — plagued by pestilence, hunger and war — were miserable old times, nor do we have a good reason for looking into the future pessimistically. Admittedly, a physiologically secure and standardised long life does not necessarily mean a fulfilled long life. Even if we take an optimistic view of the future its realisation would entail our facing immense tasks. So let us tackle them!

I, too, started out, a dozen years ago or so, with pure historical demography, decimal points, learning computer technology and its uses, statistical analysis, the epidemiology of infectious diseases, etc. The 'real questions' came much later, namely when I was asked by physicians, folklorists, theologians, psychologists, sociologists, fellow historians, students, 'ordinary people', what all my research *really* meant, why I investigated such a mass of material from parish registers and central statistical bureaux, what really changed during the last three or four hundred years with regard to death and dying, where we stand, and where we and our children and children's children are to go. The historian, then, should not stay in his ivory tower nor play number games, but meet all kinds of people, consider their questions seriously and in depth and try to find answers to them. I really think he has his duty towards society. So let us go beyond decimal points!

Notes

1. Concerning the old question about the consequences of including rural districts into an expanding city marketing region, see, for instance, the recent survey by Maurice Aymard, 'Autoconsommation et marchés: Chayanov, Labrousse ou Le Roy Ladurie?' in *Annales: E.S.C., 38* (1983), 1393–1410. Regarding the development in Nedertorneå, see the dissertation by Anders Brändström, *De kärlekslösa mödrarna. Spädbarnsdödligheten i Sverige under 1800–talet med särskild hänsyn till Nedertorne*å församling, (Stockholm, Almqvist and Wiksell, 1984), specially chapter VI.

2. 'Unterschiedliche Säuglingssterblichkeit in Deutschland, 18. bis 20. Jahrundert — Warum', *Zeitschrift für Bevölkerungswissenschaft, 7* (1981), p. 376.

3. On this see Jacques Dupâquier, 'Les progrès décisifs de la démographie', in J. Dupâquier, *Pour la démographie historique* (Paris, Presses Universitaires de France, 1984), pp. 146–9. Dupâquier here also deals with the controversy about the so-called 'urban graveyard effect' which has involved in recent years chiefly A. Sharlin, A. M. Van de Woude and A. Perrenoud.

4. One of the best studies is still, in my opinion, that by Alfred Perrenoud, 'L'inégalité sociale devant la mort à Genève au XVIIe siècle', *Population, 30* (1975), numéro spécial (Démographie historique), 211–43. See also chapter V in the thesis by Jean-Pierre Bardet: 'Le réseau social: différences et divergence', in idem: *Rouen au XVIIe et XVIIIe siècles. Les mutations d'un espace social.* (Paris, Société d'Edition d'Enseignement Superieur, 1983), pp. 225–62.

5. For a survey from the point of view of historical demography see Hector Gutierrez and Jacques Houdaille, 'La mortalité maternelle en France au XVIIIe siècle', *Population, 38* (1983), 975–94. From the point of view of medical history, H.J. Schneegans, 'Die Müttersterblichkeit im 17. bis 19. Jahrhundert', *Zentralblatt für Gynäkologie, 104* (1982), 1416–20. In Sweden Ulf Högberg of the University of Umeå is working on a comprehensive research project on the mortality of mothers in that country from 1749 to 1980. See his *Maternal mortality.* Research report, January, 1984, mimeo, Umeå, 1984. Also V. Högberg 'Mödradöd i förhistorisk tid', *Sydsvenska medicinhistoriska Sällskapets årsskrift, 20* (1983), 103–14.

6. See the article written with Geneviève Heller, 'Körperliche Über-lastung von Frauen im 19. Jahrhundert', in Arthur E. Imhof (ed.) *Der Mensch und sein Körper von der Antike bis heute* (Munich, Beck, 1983), 137–56.

7. Specific analyses on causes of death across space and time have been prominent for a long time in the earlier history of medicine. The literature is correspondingly comprehensive. For your guidance see Christa Habrich and others (eds), 'Medizinische Diagnostik in Geschichte und Gegenwart', *Festschrift für Heinz Goerke zum 60. Geburtstag* (Munich, Werner Fritsch-Verlag, 1978). On the concept of so-called pathokoinosis and its dynamism in a historical context, the principle has been explained by Mirko D. Grmek, *Les maladies à l'aube de la civilisation occidentale* (Paris, Payot, 1983), 14–17.

8. For a rapid survey see Robert Muchembled and others, *Nos ancêtres, les paysans* (Lille, Centre d'Histoire de la Région du Nord, 1983), especially the chapters by R. Muchembled, 'Le paysan face aux calamités naturelles, aux épidémies et aux guerres, du XVe au XVIIIe siècle', 104–13; 'Famille, sociabilité et relations sociales au village (XVe–XVIIIe siècle)', 120–9. François Lebrun, *Se soigner autrefois. Médecins, saints et sorciers aux XVIIe et XVIIIe siècles* (Paris, Temps Actuels, 1983). About an even earlier time from which, however, many occurrencees had their effects on the 19th and 20th century, see Aaron J. Gurjewitsch, *Das Weltbild des mittelalterlichen Menschen* (Munich, Beck, 1980), (originally Moscow, 1972).

9. The best introduction to this theme is still Philippe Ariès, *Western attitudes towards death from the Middle Ages to the present* (Baltimore, Johns Hopkins University Press, 1974). Excellent new works dealing with long periods: Michel Vovelle, *La mort et l'Occident de 1300 à nos jours* (Paris, Gallimard, 1983); and Alain Croix and Fanch Roudant *Les Bretons, la mort et Dieu de 1600 à nos jours* (Paris, Messidor/Temps Actuels, 1984). Speci-ally on urban mortality during the early part of the Modern Period: Pierre Chaunu, *La mort à Paris; XVIe, XVIIe et XVIIIe siècles* (Paris, Fayard, 1978).

10. Dorothy Watkins, 'Problems and Methods in the History of Medicine (Cambridge, 25–28 March 1985)', *Bulletin of the Society for the Social History of Medicine, 36* (1985), 61.

11. Ashish Bose, *Demography beyond decimal points*. Address by the Presi-dent of the Indian Association for the Study of Population, Tenth Annual Conference IIM, Bangalore, May 20–23, 1985 (Delhi, Central Electric Press, 1985,) 2, 18.

12. Pierre Goubert, 'Sur trois siècles et trois décennies. Passage des Mèthodologies', *Méthodologie de l'Histoire et des sciences humaines. Mèlanges en l'Honneur de Fernand Braudel,* vol. 2 (Toulouse, Privat, 1973), 256–7.

13. See my *Die Gewonnenen Jahre* (Munich, Beck, 1981); on the past in-teraction of demographic factors with people's every-day life see my *Die Verlorenen Welten* (Munich, Beck, 1984).

6

No Death Without Birth: The Implications of English Mortality in the Early Modern Period

E. A. Wrigley

It is obvious that for most of human history fertility and mortality must have been at closely similar levels. For the former to have fallen short of the latter consistently would have meant extinction, while the opposite case could not have long continued because of the impossibility of increasing food supplies other than very slowly.[1] Man is a slow-breeding animal and, therefore, human mortality was always at a far lower level than in most other animals. There is no reason to suppose that crude birth rates in any large population consistently exceeded about 50 per 1000. Equally, there can be no reason to believe that crude death rates ever significantly exceeded this level. In individual years and in exceptional circumstances far higher death rates occurred, but even when such mortality surges occurred the usual situation must have been very different. This in turn implies that expectation of life at birth can seldom have been much less than 20 years at birth, and that where this was so, the gross reproduction rate was in the range 3.0–3.5. Those women who survived to the end of the child-bearing period bore about seven children on average.[2]

An expectation of life at birth of 20 years represents a drastically more severe mortality regime than that experienced today when expectation of life at birth (e_0) is about 75 years in advanced communities, but even so it is possible to exaggerate the uncertainty of life in such circumstances. Under the age of one, and to a lesser degree under the age of five, life is desperately hazardous. More than half of each new birth cohort dies before reaching their fifth birthday. Thereafter the dangers ease. More than three-quarters of those who celebrate their fifth birthday live to see 20; and of those who see 20 almost a half also reach 50.[3] This represents a disturbing contrast with the best modern states, where over 90 per cent of each new cohort can expect to survive beyond the end of their fifth decade, compared with only about 1 in 6 where $e_0 = 20$, but one might well draw still more depressing conclusions about the uncertainty of life in the past from some of the more strongly highlighted descriptions of conditions in earlier centuries.

In any case, the same line of reasoning immediately suggests that in pre-industrial western Europe mortality took a far less heavy toll. The general warrant for this assertion lies in the wide prevalence of the 'European' marriage pattern in Europe north of the Alps and the Pyrenees and west of the Oder. The European marriage pattern was unique, so far as is known, in that the average age at first marriage for women was the mid-20s, and a significant fraction of all women who survived to the end of the child-bearing period never married. This sets a comparatively low upper level to fertility and, on the assumption that growth rates must be close to zero, implies an equally modest level of mortality. For example, if the average age at first marriage for women is 26 and 12 per cent of each cohort never marry, and assuming marital fertility levels similar to those found in England in the 17th and 18th centuries with a mean age at maternity of 32 years, it can be shown that a stationary population will result from an e_0 in women of 32.5 years.[4]

A regime of the 'European' type involves substantially less destructive mortality rates than where e_0 is 20 years. In these circumstances over 84 per cent of all 5-year-olds reach 20, and more than three-fifths of the latter reach 50. The infant mortality rate is about 220 per 1000 compared with almost 350 per 1000 in the more severe alternative. In a stationary population with these characteristics, the crude birth and death rates are about 32 per 1000. In England in the final quarter of the 17th century, when the intrinsic growth rate was close to zero, the prevailing crude birth and death rates were approximately at this level.[5]

It is well outside the scope of this essay to attempt to deal *in extenso* with the available evidence of the contrast between the 'European' demographic regime found in western Europe and that found in other parts of Europe, still less with extra-European areas. However, as an illustration of the scale of the differences between eastern and western European countries, consider the data in Table 6.1. The data in the top panel relate to the 1870s, the earliest full decade for which national registration data exist for the east European countries. Death rates in the 1870s were

Table 6.1: Crude birth and death rates (CBR and CDR, respectively) in eastern and western Europe (rates per 1000 total population).

1870–9	CBR	CDR
England and Wales	35.5	21.6
Norway	30.8	17.1
Sweden	30.4	18.4
Hungary	43.4	40.7
Russia	50.3	36.3
Serbia	40.9	34.5

	England		Norway		Sweden	
	CBR	CDR	CBR	CDR	CBR	CDR
1750–9	33.4	26.1	33.9	24.6	35.8	27.4
1760–9	34.4	28.4	34.7	27.5	34.5	27.5
1770–9	36.2	26.6	30.2	26.0	32.7	29.4
1780–9	36.7	27.7	30.3	25.5	32.5	27.1
1790–9	38.9	26.4	32.9	22.3	33.5	25.3

Sources: For all data in the top panel and for Norway and Sweden in the bottom panel, B.R. Mitchell, *European historical statistics 1750–1975*, 2nd rev. edn (London, 1981), table B6. For data for England 1750–99; Wrigley and Schofield, *Population history of England,* table A3.3, 531–4.

about twice as high in the east as in the west, and birth rates were also substantially higher. Rates of natural increase were lower in the eastern countries, except in the case of Russia where the crude birth rate exceeded 50 per 1000, an exceptional figure. Crude rates are, of course, an imperfect guide to the underlying fertility and mortality conditions, but the contrast is too marked to be attributable to differences in, say, age structure. By the 1870s some decline in mortality had already taken place in western Europe, and indeed the first signs of a secular fall in fertility were visible in places. For England, Norway and Sweden, however, crude birth and death rates are also available for the second half of the 18th century. These are set out in the lower panel of Table 6.1. Of the 15 decennial death rates for the three countries all except two lay between 25 and 30 per 1000, somewhat higher than their rates in the 1870s, but far lower than late 19th century rates in eastern Europe (the two exceptions were both in Norway, in the 1750s and 1790s). The birth rates were normally between 30 and 35, little different from their rates in the 1870s (the exceptions were England 1770–99 and Sweden 1750–9; all four cases lay between 35 and 40).

135

Using the countries for which data are reproduced in Table 6.1 may overstate the extent of the contrast between east and west. For example, crude birth and death rates in France in the later 18th century were substantially higher than in England, Norway or Sweden. Decadal birth rates between 1750–9 and 1790–9 ranged between 36.9 and 40.4 per 1000; the comparable death rates between 33.3 and 36.3.[6] In eastern Europe, too, less extreme cases may have existed. The late-19th century vital registration data suggest, for example, that birth and death rates in Rumania were lower than in Hungary, Russia or Serbia. But the contrast between western and eastern Europe was marked and the concomitants of the two regimes have wide historical importance.[7]

Since such heavy stress has often been put on the severity of mortality in the past, it is worth noting that dealing in generalities as I have just done may actually tend to convey too dark an impression even in the case of west European countries. There are two considerations that point to this conclusion so far as early modern England is concerned. First, while in the whole sweep of the historic past it is safe to assume an absence of significant population growth,[8] in early modern England it was unusually rapid, either when compared with earlier periods or with other European countries between the 16th and 19th centuries.[9] Over the quarter-millenium from 1550 to 1800 the annual rate of population growth was about 0.5 per cent per annum: at times it approached 1.0 per cent per annum. Crude birth and death rates were therefore up to 10 per 1000 per annum apart in the period. In the main the difference from the stationary situation sketched above[10] was due to the existence of higher levels of fertility than those used for purposes of illustration, but in some degree the gap arose because mortality was lower than implied by the e_0 employed to illustrate the stationary case. Expectation of life at birth was lower in the second half of the 17th century than in any other comparable period from 1550 to 1850.[11]

Second, mortality at any one time was far from uniform. There were always major regional differences. Low-lying, marshy areas, for example, were very much less healthy than well-drained uplands. More importantly, there was in general a consistent and strong relation between population density and mortality levels. Urban populations, even in market towns of a very modest size, suffered higher death rates than neighbouring rural areas. Large towns such as York, Bristol, Norwich, Newcastle or, preeminently, London, often failed to balance their demographic books. More were buried than were born within city walls and in the surrounding suburbs. Without a steady stream of immigrants many, perhaps most, towns before the 19th century would have lost population. Proximity of man to man, impure water, and the inability to remove animal and vegetable waste products, created an environment in which lethal diseases were widely prevalent. Urban mortality rates have proved difficult to measure with precision, but both the urban crude death rates, where they can be estimated, and the available information about age-specific mortality suggest that expectation of life at birth in an urban environment was frequently in the range between 20 and 35 years and sometimes below 20.[12]

The opposite side of the coin, of course, is that there were many rural areas where mortality levels were substantially better than those that result from a generalised calculation relating to the country as a whole. The proportion of the English population living in towns was very modest in Elizabethan times but rose greatly in the next 200 years. For example, if any settlement with 5,000 or more inhabitants is treated as a town, the urban percentage rose from 8 in 1600 to 28 in 1800.[13] If allowance is also made for the 'weight' of deeply unhealthy rural areas and for the existence of larger areas of relatively high mortality, it will occasion no surprise that death rates in much of the country were substantially lower than in the country as a whole.

The parish of Hartland in Devon is a good example of the modest level of mortality found where conditions were favourable in early modern England. Hartland is situated in the far northwest of Devon, remote from highways with the sea on two sides of the roughly square parish. It was a parish with a population varying between about 1,000 and 1,500, largely devoted to agriculture with many scattered farmsteads. It possesses a good parish register, which allowed a family reconstitution study to be carried out. This showed that the age-specific mortality rates up to age 15 suggest an expectation of life at birth of 55 years or more throughout the period from Elizabethan times to the beginning of Victoria's reign.[14]

Of the parishes so far reconstituted, no other has such low mortality as Hartland, but several are only marginally less favourably placed. Since it may occasion some surprise that individual parishes could boast expectation of life at birth as high in the 16th, 17th and 18th centuries as those attained nationally only about 1920, it is worth examining the considerations that suggest that the reconstitution data are tolerably accurate.

The most plausible reason for supposing mortality to have been under-estimated is that the number of deaths occurring in the parish exceeded the number recorded in its registers. If this had happened it is to be expected that it would have affected particularly the recording of the burials of young infants, especially before baptism. Once a child had been baptised, and more especially if it had survived long enough to have acquired social visibility, it is far less likely that, following death, it would not have been accorded normal burial rites and have found a place in the burial register. Infant mortality, in short, might be expected to be under-estimated more substantially than mortality at later ages. Infant mortality in Hartland was indeed very low, under 100 per 1000 in the 17th and 18th centuries, but its level was just what would be expected from the mortality rates of the age groups 1–4, 5–9 and 10–14 on the assumption that Hartland experienced a mortality regime of the type represented by model North in the Princeton regional tables.[15] In this Hartland's experience was typical of the relative levels of infant and child mortality in the great majority of English parishes. It is worth noting in this regard that *some* English reconstitutions do reveal high rates of infant and child mortality. In Gainsborough, for example, a market town of some size, infant mortality was above 250 per 1000 in the three successive 50-year periods between 1600 and 1750.[16]

Two further considerations reinforce the view that the low mortality rates found in a number of English reconstitution studies are probably broadly accurate. First, when the state established a vital registration system in 1837 the level of infant mortality found in the published tabulations was very often very low in areas where reconstitution studies had suggested low risk to infant life. For example in the Bideford and Holsworthy registration districts, of which in 1841 the parish of Hartland represented 7.0 per cent of the total population, the infant mortality rate in 1838–1844 was 97 per 1000.[17] Any under-registration of deaths in the early years of the new state system is thought to have been slight, and this was probably especially true of rural areas. Since mortality improvements in 19th-century England were modest until after 1870, the evidence drawn from the early years of state registration constitutes persuasive support for the credibility of the low infant mortality rates found for earlier periods in some reconstitution studies.[18]

Second, while the mortality rates found in west European

reconstitution studies and in other studies that use analogous methods are in general higher than those found in England, high expectations of life and very low infant and child mortality rates have been discovered in some areas. In parts of Scandinavia infant mortality rates of less than 150 per 1000 were not uncommon, and there were also parts of Germany where such rates were to be found.[19]

Two factors appear to have been especially conducive to low mortality and especially to low mortality early in life. The first has already been touched upon. High population density meant increased exposure to contact with disease carriers: low density usually led to a relative freedom from infection. The second concerns the length and intensity of breastfeeding. Where breastfeeding was brief infant mortality was high and marital fertility was also above average because of the relatively short period of amenorrhoea implied by early weaning. Where children were as a rule principally breast-fed until beyond their first birthday, infant mortality was normally much lower and birth intervals were relatively long. In England there is persuasive indirect evidence that the average duration of breastfeeding was about 15 months, a period sufficiently long to exercise an important influence in keeping infant mortality at a modest level.[20]

A number of reflections suggest themselves in the light of the foregoing.

1. While there must have been many populations in pre-industrial times that had no alternative but to seek to sustain high levels of fertility because life was short and uncertain for reasons outside their control, there may have been cases where mortality was well above the 'platform' level set by the nature of the local disease environment because fertility was high. We are familiar with the argument that where, say, malaria was widely prevalent, the local population would be obliged to accept a low expectation of life and therefore had to foster and sustain social customs such as early and universal marriage, which served to promote high fertility and so avoid a negative intrinsic growth rate and ultimate extinction. Any group that failed to act in this way would in time be replaced by one whose conventions of life were better adapted to the exigencies of the local situation. We are less accustomed to consider the possibility that the kind of social conventions well suited to coping with prevailing high levels of mortality may themselves have produced the situation to which they were well adapted when the group in question lived in an area in which

mortality was *not* necessarily at a high overall level. This was the kind of circumstance that Malthus had in mind in referring to a 'Chinese' situation, where population was 'forced'.[21]

The two possible situations are not symmetric. If a population in an area in which environmental influences imposed high mortality failed to produce large families it would die out. If a population, living in an area in which the range and types of local diseases and of other environmental influences on mortality implied a much lower level of minimum mortality, had a higher level of fertility than was 'necessary', it would not necessarily disappear, or fail to survive for other reasons, though it might be condemned to lower living standards and harsher conditions of life than would otherwise be necessary because mortality had risen to match fertility and population totals were larger than would otherwise have been the case.

The matter can be set out diagrammatically. In Figure 6.1(a) the background level of mortality is high, because, say, of the prevalence of insect-borne and parasitic diseases. It is a condition for the successful continuation of population in the area that fertility should match this level. It might perhaps be called the 'West African' situation. (In all the diagrams in Figure 6.1 the levels of fertility and mortality shown are intended to capture long-term trends only: they do not therefore reflect the likelihood of notable, and, in the case of mortality, occasionally violent short-term fluctuation.) In Figure 6.1(b) we have the 'Chinese' case. The background level of mortality is far lower but fertility is high and invariant, because, say, by social convention all women on or before reaching sexual maturity must be married and are therefore at risk to bear children throughout their fertile lives (though conventions about remarriage may modify this generalisation somewhat). Figure 6.1(c) relates to a third possibility, the west European case. The mortality graph reproduces the curve of 6.1(b), that is we assume that the background level of mortality and the response of mortality to increasing population pressure are the same in both cases. Fertility, however, is lower, because women marry eight to ten years after menarche rather than in rough coincidence with it, and also because a substantial fraction of each cohort, ranging from a tenth up to a fifth or even a quarter, never marry. The mere fact of a lower level of fertility ensures that population growth will cease at a lower total than in 6.1(b); the situation is inherently less 'forced'. But if fertility is also responsive to increasing population pressure, as shown in the

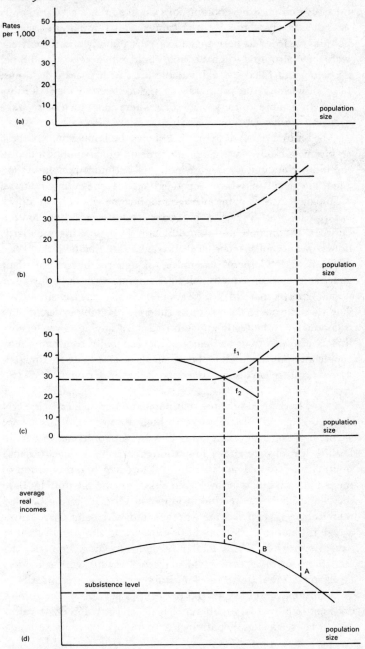

*Figure 6.1: Fertility, mortality and living standards. —, fertility; ▬,
mortality.*

f_2 variant, population growth will cease at a still-earlier point, perhaps when mortality is scarcely higher than its platform level. Such a situation would obtain, for example, if in a predominantly peasant society there were a conventional minimum size of holding regarded as necessary to sustain a family and if marriage were only permitted when a couple could gain access to a holding. As settlement filled the cultivatable area with peasant holdings, nuptiality would be progressively reduced and with it fertility also.[22] In a more complex economy where most men were wage earners, similar arrestor mechanisms might also exist.[23]

The bottom panel of Figure 6.1 shows the implications of these several possibilities for living standards on the assumption that in pre-industrial circumstances a notional optimum population existed, the level of which depended on the prevailing material technology. At this point average real income would be at a peak unattainable at higher population totals, where the tension between production and reproduction pushes living standards down towards subsistence level. It will be seen that both the 'West African' and 'Chinese' examples, though so different in their genesis, result in equally bleak economic prospects for their populations (A in 6.1(d)): they are both 'high-pressure' situations. The west European case is quite different. Having lower fertility is conducive to better living standards (B); having lower fertility that is also sensitive to deteriorating economic conditions may enable an optimum state to be attained, or closely approximated, a 'low-pressure' solution at the opposite extreme from the first two types (C).

2. We have already noted that population growth rates in early modern England were remarkably high. At first sight this is very surprising, since nuptiality was low and in consequence overall fertility was also generally low, though variable in level because nuptiality fluctuated considerably.[24] Moreover, the proportion of the population living in towns and cities rose rapidly until by 1800 the Netherlands was the only country in Europe more urbanised than England, yet urban life was most unhealthy and *ceteris paribus* a high urban proportion might be expected to slow rather than to expedite growth.[25] As a matter of demographic arithmetic, the fact that growth rates were high though fertility was at modest levels implies that death rates must have been low. Admittedly, a growth rate averaging only 0.5 per cent (5 per 1000), per annum does not require a large difference between birth and death rates, but it may seem slightly paradoxical that modest fertility and high

growth rates should have gone hand in hand. Further reflection suggests a different reaction. A 'low pressure' demographic system such as England had may not only benefit individuals at any given level of population by ensuring that there is less tension between numbers and the resources available for their support than under a 'high pressure' regime, but may also facilitate more rapid long-term growth. It is not difficult to appreciate the potential advantage of a 'low pressure' system in terms of an equilibrium, or static situation, such as that illustrated in Figure 6.1.

At a given level of material technology, a population with the characteristics of f_2 in Figure 6.1(c) will be smaller than populations of the 6.1(a) or 6.1(b) types, but it may none the less enjoy greater potential for growth if it is the case that the higher current level of real incomes stimulates demand for products and services beyond the basic necessities of life, and so fosters developments in secondary and tertiary industry that would otherwise be absent. Primary industry, too, may benefit, for example as a result of the growth in towns brought about by the growing scale and changing structure of demand.[26] The significance of low mortality, in other words, may go well beyond the simple arithmetic fact that low death rates make relatively high growth rates easier to obtain. The absence of low mortality does not just have a bearing on the question of growth in demographic terms: it may also be a symptom of an economic, social or wider environmental context in which the development of the economy in ways likely to encourage growth is difficult or impossible.

3. Improved knowledge of mortality levels in pre-industrial England also throws a new light on changes in more recent periods. When McKeown showed that specific medical therapy appears to have made only a limited contribution to the fall in mortality before about 1930, even though the fall had been in train for at least 80 years, it occasioned some surprise.[27] In part the surprise probably reflected the belief that by the early 20th century expectation of life at birth was at a far higher level than any prevailing in earlier centuries. As an observation applied to the national entity, the supposition was justified, but inasmuch as remarkably modest mortality prevailed in some communities three or four centuries ago, and perhaps earlier, any surprise may have been misplaced. The reasons for the fall in mortality in the second half of the 19th century are still not well understood and it would therefore be absurd to press any parallel with earlier times, but the mere knowledge that expectations of life at birth of

about 50 years were found in some places in earlier periods puts the later 19th century and early 20th centuries in a new perspective.

An adequate level of nutrition, a tolerably pure water supply, a fairly low level of contact with serious infectious disease and an absence of opportunities for the rapid multiplication of disease vectors, such as those afforded by putrescent animal or vegetable wastes, may permit an average life span of half a century even though medical knowledge is slight and medical practitioners may be few and ignorant. Such conditions may arise, as in the case of Hartland, from a combination of remoteness, light population density, and a relatively favourable ratio of agricultural land to mouths in need of food. Equally, the increased wealth of a country that has undergone an industrial revolution may secure the same advantages even for crowded city populations by investment in water supply and sewage systems, combined with cheap transport to link urbanised populations to distant food supplies, and the enforcement by governments of quarantine regulations and by families and local communities of isolation rules for individuals suffering from infectious ailments. Such changes, helped by cheap fuel for domestic heating, more thorough cooking and more convenient cleansing of clothes and persons, were evidently capable of securing substantial improvements in mortality since comparable circumstances arising for different reasons had led to broadly similar low mortality in much earlier times.

Recognition of the immense significance of the west European marriage pattern has transformed work on population history in recent years. It has proved as important for family history, for the study of household composition, for understanding systems of property transmission between the generations, for grasping the significance of the institution of service, and even for certain aspects of economic history, as for understanding the history of nuptiality and fertility.[28] Perhaps, however, its importance for the understanding of the history of mortality has been too little stressed.

The European marriage system is a 'luxury' that populations through much of the traditional world may have been unable to afford. Where endemic diseases were many and fatal, where epidemic diseases were frequent and devastating, where food supplies were subject to violent and unpredictable fluctuations, or where some combination of these dangers prevailed, early and universal marriage may have been mandatory. Only if a fairly long life-span is attainable is a modest level of fertility feasible, such as must follow from the practice of late marriage and frequent celibacy. It would be rash, however, to assume that only in western Europe were the disease environment and agricultural practices such that the platform level of mortality was low. The issue is not capable of demonstration, at least in the present state of knowledge, but it is likely that mortality regimes were frequently 'manufactured' by the social customs, which exercised such a strong influence on fertility levels, and thus indirectly on mortality. Societies that placed a premium on early marriage and high fertility were thereby unwittingly also placing an equal premium on high mortality.[29]

The same point can be made in a different way. If marriage had been early and universal in England and therefore fertility high, there can be no doubt that mortality would have been equally high, or virtually so. In one sense, therefore, the low level of death rates in early modern England was the gift of the marriage practices of the day. They were a necessary if not a sufficient condition of low mortality.

It is more than simply a platitude to remark that death is the inevitable consequence of birth. How early death followed birth was, of course, much influenced by the types of disease prevalent in a community; by the extent of social knowledge of ways of treating, avoiding or preventing disease; by a host of social customs that affected the probability of contracting and combatting disease;[30] and by economic conditions. But the average lapse of time between birth and death was also conditioned by the intensity of fertility in the population. High birth rates could not fail, in most traditional societies, to be matched by equally high death rates, or, in other words, by a brief interval between birth and death. Causation might run either way between the two, or in both directions. The same was true of low rates in the two categories.

Accurate information is scarce or non-existent for most countries. Enough has been learned in the last 40 years to have overturned much of the received wisdom about population history, and to encourage speculation, but far more information would be a welcome aid in separating the wheat from the chaff in current theorising. In that spirit it is reasonable to suggest, though difficult to prove (in either the older or newer sense of the word) that, in seeking to understand the notably modest level of mortality in early modern England, one should look as much to the circumstances of birth as to those of death.

Notes

1. This generalisation is true only if migration is ignored. For very large units of area or population this is a defensible simplification. In small units, however, relatively large net migration balances may be a longstanding feature of the local situation, and may vitiate the generalisation.

2. These results follow from stable population theory given that crude birth and death rates were at the level suggested and in the absence of any significant natural increase or decrease.

3. These data were derived from the Princeton model North life tables, combining the l_x values for the two sexes. The information used in constructing these tables all related to 19th or 20th century populations. More severe levels of mortality than those experienced in the recent past were extrapolated from the material available. In general, however, this does not appear to have led to inaccuracy. Mortality studies of populations living in earlier periods, for example reconstitution studies using parish registers, normally produce patterns of age-specific mortality rates that conform quite closely to model life tables. There is one important exception to this generalisation, however. The model life table death rates for women in the child-bearing groups are usually similar to those for men, or even somewhat lower, but maternal death rates in the past were high enough at times to suggest that female mortality, among married women at least, may be understated in model life tables. A.J. Coale and P. Demeny, *Regional model life tables and stable populations* (Princeton, 1966). See also 15, below. On maternal mortality, see R.S. Schofield, 'Did the mothers really die? Three centuries of maternal mortality in "The World we have lost"' in L. Bonfield, R.M. Smith and K. Wrightson (eds), *The world we have gained* (Oxford, 1986), 231–60.

4. The age-specific marital fertility rates used in this illustrative calculation for the five-year age groups 25–9 to 45–9 were 360, 300, 250, 130 and 30 per 1000. With a mean age of marriage of 26 years, this implies that the average married woman surviving to the end of the childbearing period would have 4.99 children, of which, assuming a sex ratio at birth of 105:100, 2.43 would be female. Allowing for the assumption that 12 per cent of women never marry (and assuming, unrealistically, that there is no illegitimate fertility), the figure of 2.43 for married women is reduced to 2.14 for all women. And it will be found that the proportion of women surviving to the mean age at maternity in the model North life tables, to which English mortality in the early modern period conformed fairly closely, is such as to imply, with an expectation of life at birth of 32.5 years, that each generation of women were replaced by an equal number in the next generation. For a fuller discussion of the method and assumptions used, with more elaborate model calculations, see E.A. Wrigley and R.S. Schofield, *The population history of England. A reconstruction* (London, 1981), 265–9.

5. They were 31.2 and 30.3, respectively, averaged over 5 quinquennia from 1674–8 to 1694–8. Wrigley and Schofield, *Population History of England,* table A3.1, 528–9.

6. L. Henry and Y. Blayo, 'La population de la France de 1740 à 1860', *Population*, numéro spécial, *30* (1975), table 22, 109.

7. For works dealing with various aspects of the wider issues see 28, below.

8. Or more precisely a rate of growth so slight on average that the demographic characteristics of the population in question must have been barely distinguishable from those of a stationary population.

9. There are estimates of population totals and population growth rates for all the main west European countries between the mid-16th and early 19th centuries in E.A. Wrigley, 'The growth of population in eighteenth-century England: a conundrum resolved', *Past and Present, 98* (1983), 121–50.

10. P. 134.

11. Detailed information about English crude birth and death rates, gross and net reproduction rates, and expectation of life at birth between 1541 and 1871 may be found in Wrigley and Schofield, *Population history of England,* appendix 3, 527–35.

12. On the unhealthiness of marshy areas generally, and the especially acute problems of malarial areas, see M.J. Dobson, 'Population, disease and mortality in southeast England, 1600–1800' (unpub. D. Phil. thesis, Oxford, 1982), chapters 8 and 9, 'The unhealthy marshlands', and 'Mosquitoes and malaria'.

The literature on urban mortality is enormous. Two issues of *Annales de démographie historique*, those of 1978 and 1962, contained substantial sections with a variety of articles on the subject (the sections entitled 'Etudes de mortalité' and 'Villes du passé', respectively). Similarly, J. Meyer, A. Lottin, J.P. Poussou, H. Soly, B. Vogler and A. van der Woude, *Etudes sur les villes en Europe occidentale, milieu du XVIIe siècle à la veille de la révolution française,* 2 vols (Paris, 1983) contains some substantive discussion and much bibliographical material. An important new aspect to the discussion of the issue of urban mortality was opened by A. Sharlin, 'Natural decrease in early modern cities: a reconsideration', *Past and Present, 79* (1978), 126–38. But see R. Finlay, 'Natural decrease in early modern cities', *Past and Present, 92* (1981), 169–74; and A.M. van der Woude, 'Population developments in the northern Netherlands (1500–1800) and the validity of the ''urban graveyard'' effect', *Annales de démographie historique* (1982), 55–75.

13. E.A. Wrigley, 'Urban growth and agricultural change: England and the continent in the early modern period', *Journal of Interdisciplinary History, XV* (1985), table 2, 688.

14. The surviving Hartland parish registers begin in 1558. The family reconstitution exercise was carried down to 1837, the date of inception of a state system of vital registration. The logic of family reconstitution is such that age-specific mortality can be most accurately measured for children up to the age at which they leave home. Estimates of e_0 derived only from death rates up to age 15, however, are unlikely to be subject to wide margins of error because the shape of the mortality curve above 15 years is closely related to its shape below that age. The proportions surviving from birth to age 15, l_{15}, for the successive half-centuries 1600–49 to 1750–99, were 830, 832, 791 and 871.

15. The model North tables were based on Swedish mortality data between 1851 and 1890 (4 tables), Norwegian data between 1856 and 1880, and again between 1946 and 1955 (4 tables), and an Icelandic life table for 1941–50. Coale and Dimeny, *Regional model life tables,* 14. Evidence of the good fit between infant mortality rates and the rates for the age groups 1–4, 5–9 and 10–14 in Hartland may be found in E.A. Wrigley and R.S. Schofield, 'English population history from family reconstitution: summary results 1600–1799', *Population Studies, 37* (1983), table 14, 179, and more generally 175–80.

16. Wrigley and Schofield, 'English population history from family reconstitution', table 14, p. 179.

17. *Ninth Annual Report of the Registrar General* (London, 1849), 214. The combined population of the two registration districts in 1841 was 31,934; of Hartland 2,223.

18. The absence of any substantial improvement in expectation of life at birth in the country as a whole before 1870 may be deceptive. There were probably favourable changes in mortality rates in most types of community but compositional shifts in the population were increasing the proportion living in the least healthy areas as the populations of the cities grew rapidly. For an illuminating discussion of the issue, see R. Woods, 'The effects of population redistribution on the level of mortality in nineteenth-century England and Wales', *Journal of Economic History, xlv* (1985), 645–51.

19. For Scandinavia, for example, A. Brändström and J. Sundin, 'Infant mortality in a changing society. The effects of child care in a Swedish parish 1820–1894', in A. Brändström and J. Sundin (eds.), *Tradition and transition.* Studies in microdemography and social change, no. 2 (Umeå, 1981), 67–104; O. Turpeinen, 'Infant mortality in Finland 1749–1865', *Scandinavian Economic History Review, xxvii* (1979), 1–21: for Germany, A.E. Imhof, 'Unterschiedliche Säuglingssterblichkeit in Deutschland, 18. bis. 20. Jahrhundert — warum?', *Zeitschrift for Bevölkerungswissenschaft, 7* (1981), 343–82, and Imhof, 'The amazing simultaneousness of the big differences and the boom on the nineteenth century — some facts and hypotheses about infant and maternal mortality in Germany, eighteenth to twentieth century', in T. Bengtsson, G. Fridlizius, and R. Ohlsson (eds), *Pre-industrial population change, the mortality decline and short-term population movements* (Stockholm, 1984), 191–222. Knodel also identifies some parishes, such as Werdum, where infant mortality was very low. J. Knodel, 'Natural fertility in pre-industrial Germany', *Population Studies, xxxii* (1978), 481–510. Low rates may also be found in individual parishes in countries where infant mortality was generally high. For example, in France Galliano's study of 18 parishes near Paris shows that the general level of infant mortality during the period 1774–1794 was fairly high (177 per 1,000) but in Le Plessis, Chevilly, Thiais and Montrouge the rates were 123, 124, 135 and 139 per 1,000, respectively. P. Galliano, 'La mortalité infantile dans le banlieue sud de Paris à la fin du XVIIIe siècle (1774–1794)', *Annales de démographie historique* (1966), table 1, 146–7.

20. Knodel's classic study of three Bavarian villages in the later 19th century showed the striking differences obtaining between places where babies were weaned at birth and those where breastfeeding over six

months or more was normal. In Schonberg and Anhausen infant mortality (including stillbirths) was about 400 per 1,000 births (including stillbirths); in Mommlingen about 170. The effect on fertility was also dramatic. Birth intervals in Mommlingen were almost a year longer than in the other two parishes in cases where the preceding child survived. J. Knodel, 'Infant mortality and fertility in three Bavarian villages: an analysis of family histories from the nineteenth century', *Population Studies, xxii* (1968), 297–318. For the estimation of the average duration of breastfeeding in pre-industrial England, see C. Wilson, 'Marital fertility in pre-industrial England, 1550–1849' (unpub. Ph.D. thesis, Cambridge, 1982), chapter 8, 'Post-partum non susceptibility', 135–54. There is an excellent review of many topics related to breastfeeding and much fascinating empirical data in C. Vandenbroeke, F. van Poppel and A. van der Woude, 'De zuigelingen- en kindersterfte in Belgie end Nederland in seculair perspectief', *Tijdschrift voor Geschiedenis, 94* (1981), 461–91.

21. T.R. Malthus, *An essay on the principle of population* (London, 1798), 129–31.

22. See G. Ohlin, 'Mortality, marriage and population growth in pre-industrial populations', *Population Studies, xiv* (1961), 190–7; and R.S. Schofield, 'The relationship between demographic structure and environment in pre-industrial western Europe', in W. Conze (ed.), *Sozialgeschichte der Familie in der Neuzeit Europas* (Stuttgart, 1976), 147–60.

23. Malthus discussed this point at length on several occasions. There is an especially interesting analysis of the way in which, in a capitalist economy where most men are wage earners, market mechanisms tend to arrest population growth well before extreme destitution prevails, in T.R. Malthus, *An essay on the principle of population,* 6th edn, 2 vols, (London, 1826), book iii, chapter x, 'Of systems of agriculture and commerce combined'.

24. For two recent discussions of the evidence for fertility and nuptiality fluctuations in England between the 16th and 19th centuries, see D. Weir, 'Rather never than late: celibacy and age at marriage in English cohort fertility, 1541–1871', *Journal of Family History, 9* (1984), 341–55; and R. Schofield, 'English marriage patterns revisited', *Journal of Family History, 10* (1985), 2–20.

25. This is, however, a matter of great complexity. For interesting reflections on this and some cognate issues see J. de Vries, *European urbanization 1500–1800* (Cambridge, Mass., 1984), esp. chapter 10, 'Migration and urban growth', and the articles of Sharlin and van der Woude listed in 12, above.

26. The classic description of the beneficial possibilities of a positive feedback situation of this type remains that provided by Adam Smith, *An inquiry into the nature and causes of the wealth of nations,* ed. E. Cannan, 2 vols, 6th edn (London, 1961), i, book iii, 'Of the different progress of opulence in different nations'.

27. T. McKeown and R.G. Record, 'Reasons for the decline of mortality in England and Wales during the nineteenth century', *Population Studies, xvi* (1962), 94–122; T. McKeown, R.G. Record and R.D. Turner, 'An interpretation of the decline of mortality in England and Wales during the twentieth century', *Population Studies, xxix* (1975), 391–422.

28. See especially, J. Hajnal, 'European marriage patterns in perspective', in D. V. Glass and D.E.C. Eversley (eds.), *Population in History* (London, 1965), 101–143; P. Laslett (ed.), *Household and family in past time* (Cambridge, 1972); R. Wall (ed.), *Family forms in historic Europe* (Cambridge, 1983): R.M. Smith (ed.), *Land, kinship and life-cycle* (Cambridge, 1985); A. Kussmaul, *Servants in husbandry in early modern England* (Cambridge, 1981); and Wrigley and Schofield, *Population history of England*. The list could be very much extended, but a substantial part of the literature available may be found in the bibliographies of these works.

29. This was a point much stressed by Malthus. For example, in the course of a discussion of the degree of regularity in the paired relationships possible in the triad of births, marriages and deaths, he remarked, 'The most general rule that can be laid down on this subject is, perhaps, that any *direct* encouragement to marriage must be accompanied by an increased mortality.' He meant, of course, that the births occurring as a result would mostly fail to survive. Malthus, *Principles of population*, 6th edn, i, p. 329.

30. Probably the most important single social custom influencing mortality was the set of conventions determining the length of breastfeeding and weaning practices. But dietary conventions and taboos; personal and social hygiene; the scope, frequency and nature of migratory movements, trade and communications; prevailing customs about the scale and usage of space within dwellings; and a host of other such factors also played a part in raising or reducing susceptibility to disease and accident.

III

Computers and the History of Institutions

7

Quantitative and Qualitative Perspectives on the Asylum

Anne Digby

'Let me not be mad!' pleads King Lear when torn adrift from familiar circumstances. A semi-numerate historian, more used to qualitative methods, felt similar feelings when faced with the problems of deciding which categories of data on madness were appropriate to select for computation, enduring the ensuing tedium of preparing numerically accurate data sets, and experiencing the headaches of evaluating the results of simple computing exercises, and relating these to other sources.[1] Why then might a social historian of medicine embark on a quantitative exploration of past aspects of a mental institution to complement an investigation using more traditional qualitative methods? The main advantages appeared to be: a gain in precision in researching some key issues; an improved ability to construct a dynamic rather than a static view of an institution; and new insights not easily acquired by more traditional methods of analysis.

The Retreat and quantification

It may be helpful to suggest why the Quaker Retreat at York was thought to be of sufficient historical importance for this case-study to be worthwhile. The asylum had opened in 1796 at a time when milder methods of treating the mentally ill were being seen as both desirable and practicable. In 1813 had come the publication of the first full-length book depicting the practicalities of using these methods in an asylum; this was Samuel Tuke's *Description of the Retreat*. The book placed the Retreat in the public mind as a progressive institution, its name became identified with the mild methods of moral treatment, and a stream of visitors came there from all over the United Kingdom, western Europe, and the eastern part of the USA. The Retreat's methods were widely imitated in the asylums that were being created in such large numbers in the early part of the 19th century. A mid-19th century reformer summarised its achievement as having 'removed the final justification for neglect, brutality and crude medical methods. It proved that kindness was more effective than rigorous confinement.'[2]

After the mid-19th century the Retreat became rather a symbol of historical achievement than a current model in the world of asylumdom. And modern commentators have reflected this in dealing exclusively with the institution's earlier years. It seemed interesting to work on the Retreat's neglected archives not only to test the validity of its early reputation against its actual practice, but also to see what kind of institution it later became. Another reason for attempting a more detailed, quantitative analysis was that large hypotheses were being constructed about past asylums on the basis of little data.[3] Those who had attempted to remedy this had done so either by using small samples of patients (as a response to the large numbers of inmates in public asylums), or by analysing the total asylum population over relatively short periods of time (a response to the availability of sources). The Retreat was an ideal subject for a fuller investigation since the number of patients was relatively small by computer standards (only 2,011 patients were admitted during our period), and its archives were exceptionally detailed and continuous.

Computation seemed one obvious method of processing the large amount of data that it was possible to extract from the Retreat's archives. These went back to the opening of the asylum in 1796 and were in many instances continuous for long periods thereafter, although becoming increasingly fragmentary by the turn of the 20th century. The principal sources used for these quantitative analyses were: the admissions certificates (a complete series except for some missing ones in the early years and a lost volume for 1908); admissions registers spanning the period from 1796 to 1879; a series of seventeen medical case books from the 1790s to the 1890s; and a useful summary volume giving from 1796 to 1910 a chronological survey of patients admitted, fees paid, and duration of stay.[4]

The topics chosen for quantification covered both social and medical aspects of the asylum. Social areas investigated included changes in the composition of the patient body, in religious affiliation, gender, marital status, age, geographical origins, occupational class, fees paid, and the person or organisation sending the individual to the asylum. Medical subjects analysed included causes of mental disorder, type of illness, duration of stay, outcomes and re-admissions. Since it was intended that the analysis would help in constructing a dynamic profile of the asylum, the computer was programmed to give frequency distributions for these topics for six sub-periods within an overall period from 1796 to 1910. These sub-periods comprised the respective tenures of the Retreat's superintendents: Jepson, Allis, Thurnam, Baker, Kitching and Pierce. The data were also cross-classified in a number of ways: two of the more fruitful, as we shall see later, were to cross-tabulate varied social characteristics of patients by their religious affiliation and by their gender. Two features of the quantification deserve special emphasis. First, the methods used were all very elementary. For reasons discussed later it was thought inappropriate to adopt regression analysis or other more elaborate techniques, and the calculations consisted mostly of averages and proportions. The role of the computer was thus to handle a large data set, not to perform complex manipulations. Secondly, the ability to use a computer in this way made it unnecessary to resort to sampling. All statements relate to the complete population of the Retreat at any date (or for any period), and there is thus no question of statistical significance in relation to, say, differences of means or proportions.

Once the data had been organised the ensuing flexibility in the types of questions that could be probed with little additional effort gave a freedom and versatility to the research that would have been virtually impossible to achieve by any other route. The price that had to be paid for this euphoria was the time-consuming preparation of material into machine-readable form. In this process a major problem was in identifying the actual population to be analysed. Asylums kept their records in the form of cases in which each time an individual entered the institution he or she was given a new case number. Since patients were frequently re-admitted to the Retreat it was a lengthy task to attempt to construct a history of treatment for each individual and thus to convert cases into patients. This problem assumed large proportions since this Quaker asylum was exceptional in that its patients tended to return to it for any further period of treatment that was necessary. Tracking patients down in the records — when more than one in ten were admitted twice, and the occasional patient reappeared as many as seven, nine, thirteen or even nineteen times — was a laborious task. Fortunately, the social background of patients was very well documented so that even when re-admissions were not explicitly referred to, individuals could be identified with some degree of confidence. As a result of this tedious analysis, the 2,525 cases admitted from 1796 to 1910 were 'reconstituted' as 2,011 patients.

Two methods of organising the data set were used and each used the same subperiods in attempting to throw light on the changes that were taking place in the asylum. The first analysed first admissions in each era; this had the advantage of including all patients and of counting them only once. (It was supplemented by smaller studies of second and third admissions.) The second basic approach was to employ an analysis of patients in the Retreat at particular census dates so as to clarify differences in patient composition. Years when there was a change of superintendent were chosen because these gave both an endpoint from which to review the evolution of an earlier era, and a starting point from which to begin an assessment of developments in later years. The two approaches were complementary. The 'time series' analysis of first admissions emphasised the changes that were taking place in the flows into the Retreat during the sub-periods, while the 'census' enquiry highlighted certain features of the total asylum population at key dates. (The distinction is analogous to the more familiar treatment of births and populations in demographic studies.)

Historical insights from computing Retreat data

Detailed results of these computer analyses have been published elsewhere but it is useful here to discuss some of the more interesting findings.[5] Three central questions are explored in this section of the paper. Using the survey of first admissions the extent to which the Retreat remained Quaker in patient composition is examined, as is also the degree to which there was gender differentiation in the social and medical characteristics of patients. And using the data for selected census dates there is an analysis of whether the establishment silted up with chronic cases as contemporaries alleged was happening to the Victorian asylum.

What were the implications for the distinctive character of the York Retreat of the significant decision in 1818 to admit non-

Quaker patients to what had formerly been an entirely Quaker institution? These issues are approached through analysing first the social, and then the medical, characteristics of first admissions. The age structure of these first admissions revealed a continued 'bunching' in middle age and young adulthood, a feature also found in other Victorian mental institutions for which comparable data are available.[6] However, it was interesting to find that the concentration was less pronounced for Quaker than for non-Quaker patients; only 56 per cent of the former compared to 70 per cent of the latter were admitted in the 25 to 54 age range. As in many other 19th-century asylums, the single outnumbered the married at the Retreat. This disparity lessened during our period, largely because of a declining proportion of patients from the Society of Friends, where restrictive marriage regulations had contributed to an unusually high number of single members. In this context it is interesting to find that among the Retreat's Quaker patients 62 per cent were single compared with 50 per cent among non-Quakers, while only 27 per cent of the former were married compared with 39 per cent of the latter.

Other major changes in the social character of the asylum also came about as the result of the decision to admit non-Quakers. This not only affected the religion of first admissions but also distribution of occupational class and geographical origins. Under the first superintendent, George Jepson (1796–1823), 95 per cent of the first admissions were either members, or were connected with, the Society of Friends, whereas by the time of Bedford Pierce (1892–1910), these formed only 26 per cent of the total.[7] Non-Quaker patients first entered the asylum in 1820; the rationale for this change of policy was as a means to fulfil its charitable objectives so that the high fees paid by non-Quakers would subsidise the uneconomic contributions made by poorer Friends. This change in religious composition had interesting secondary consequences in altering the geographical areas from which patients were recruited. In the early years patients came from all over the United Kingdom, and only one-quarter were recruited from Yorkshire, but at the end of our period as many as 54 per cent came from Yorkshire, and a further 30 per cent from counties nearby. The Retreat had ceased to be a national institution and became a regional one, thus approximating to the more usual Victorian and Edwardian pattern of local recruitment to mental institutions. Yet it is interesting to note that the geographical origins of its Quaker clientele remained national not local: over the whole period there was a striking contrast between Quakers (only 24 per cent of whom came from Yorkshire) and non-Quakers (of whom 61 per cent came from there).

Associated with this increased reliance on an affluent local clientele of first admissions who were not members of the Society of Friends, was a transformation in their occupational class. In fact the Retreat increasingly approximated to its historiographical stereotype as a bourgeois institution, with a class distribution skewed to upper and middle class patients. This contrasted with its early years under Jepson when 27 per cent of first admissions came from skilled or semi-skilled occupations, and a further 12 per cent from unskilled ones. Again, this alteration was the result of the long-term adulteration of the Quaker composition of the asylum. A comparison of the occupational class of all Quaker patients with their non-Quaker counterparts gives a very different profile. Among those who were not Friends 66.1 per cent came from class 1 (gentlemen, bankers, merchants, landowners, professional men); 31.8 per cent from class 2 (retailers, teachers, craftsmen, clerks); and only 2.1 per cent from skilled, semi-skilled and non-skilled occupations.[8] In contrast, the occupational profile was more evenly divided among Friends, where 24.6 per cent came from class 1, 48.9 per cent from class 2, 18.9 per cent from class 3 (skilled or semi-skilled backgrounds), and 7.6 per cent from class 4 (unskilled occupations).

This brief review of the social character of the Retreat's first admissions suggests discontinuities rather than continuities. The picture given in 1813 in Tuke's *Description of the Retreat* was apparently increasingly falsified by events. Yet there was an interesting paradox involved in these changes. The asylum appeared to change from a national institution recruiting Quaker patients with varied occupational backgrounds to a local institution where upper and middle class patients of non-Quaker background predominated. Yet within this was a hidden kernel — almost a second asylum — where a minority of Quaker patients retained much the same social character as their predecessors had done a century before. The character of these two quite distinctive asylum populations could only have been defined by computation given the large amounts of data that needed to be cross-tabulated. We now turn to the medical records to see whether this differentiation between Quaker and non-Quaker patients was also evident in their relative duration of treatment and the outcomes of such therapy.

The Retreat's patients experienced slightly longer periods of treatment than was the case at other asylums. At York nearly half of first admissions — 49.8 per cent — stayed less than a year and a further 14.7 per cent had been discharged within the next year. On the other hand this may suggest less successful therapy or a more cautious evaluation of it by the Retreat's therapist, on the other it may plausibly suggest that financial pressures were less since many patients did not pay the economic cost of their treatment. In this context it is relevant to notice that 50.4 per cent of those paying normal fees were discharged within a year compared with only 40.6 per cent of those on subsidised terms. Since the subsidised patients were almost invariably Quakers it followed that their duration of stay was longer: only 42.6 per cent of Quaker patients emerged from the asylum within a year compared to 58.2 per cent of non-Quakers.

Closely related to periods of therapy were the outcomes of treatment. Our attention here is confined to the most favourable outcomes — those designated as 'recovered' and those labelled interchangeably as 'relieved' or 'improved'. As many as 41.2 per cent of Quakers but only 31.2 per cent of non-Quakers were said to have 'recovered'; conversely only 12.3 per cent of Quakers but 25.3 per cent of non-Quakers were said to have been 'relieved' or 'improved'. It is tempting to conclude from this that Quaker therapists were most successful at treating patients who shared the same attitudes and values. But an alternative explanation is also persuasive. Since those in the relieved category were usually those whom friends or relatives took home a little prematurely (before doctors were satisfied that convalescence was over), it is likely that financial pressures to terminate treatment were present for more non-Quaker than Quaker patients. It is also relevant to notice that recovery rates (whatever these mean!), were higher in the early than later years of the Retreat, and that this would influence the higher overall recovery rates of Quaker patients, who predominated in the earlier period.

The more problematical nature of medical records has been exemplified in this discussion of outcomes and durations of treatment. Quantitative methods in processing medical data do not necessarily overcome, and may merely make more obvious, the difficulty of framing a satisfactory interpretation of the evidence. Here, the evidence on the Retreat's durations and outcomes of treatment indicated a quite different profile of Quaker and non-Quaker patients within the same asylum, although explanations for this divergence could only be speculative.

Was the profile of women patients equally distinctive? Given that all women have tended hitherto to be hidden from history, the character of those living within the asylum has been even more obscure. It seemed worthwhile to see whether cross-tabulations could help pierce the darkness of our ignorance and perhaps qualify such simplistic images that we do possess of the female mental patient. Whether derived from contemporary assertions or recent feminist historiography these portray her as victim in one of three roles.[9] On the first of these — women whose independence and rebellion against contemporary social constraints was construed as mental illness — there is relatively little evidence. About the two other categories — those whose reproductive physiology made them peculiarly liable to mental shipwreck or those wives wrongfully and indefinitely confined because of vengeful or avaricious husbands — the Retreat data permits some useful qualifications to this impressionism.

Let us begin by looking at the general context of gender ratios at the Retreat. In the first half-century of its existence women formed about half of the patients but by the early 20th century three-fifths of the inmates were women. This situation differed from that of most other *private* mental institutions and arose both from the predominance of women over men in the Society of Friends and also the availability of subsidised terms for Quaker patients from which a disproportionate number of women benefitted. In its gender ratios the Retreat was analogous to *public,* rate-aided asylums where pauper women also outnumbered men to an increasing extent. More and more the Retreat's patients were drawn from the wider community beyond the Society of Friends. But because of the non-subsidised nature of treatment for non-Quakers, this was slightly less evident for women than for men — by the turn of the 20th century 73 per cent of women admitted but 76 per cent of men were non-Quakers.

Why and when were women sent to the Retreat? Computer analysis of the alleged causes of insanity on women's certificates by their relatives and doctors before admission gives some indication. Unfortunately, this evidence is highly problematic — as a later discussion in this essay suggests — so that little weight can be placed on precise, as opposed to general, findings. For our purposes here certain broad trends are sufficiently clear and unambiguous to be acceptable as evidence. The causes alleged for women tended increasingly to stress physical factors, whereas for men psychological factors were progressively more obvious. At the turn of the 19th century one-third of female admissions were interpreted in terms of a physical causation of insanity as against one-half a century later. In this the Retreat certificates reflected a growing emphasis in psychiatric (and gynaecological) literature on the link between the complexities of the female reproductive system and ensuing insanities of pregnancy, childbirth, lactation and menopause.[10] Qualitative analysis of some detailed submissions in later certificates confirms to some extent this view of the vulnerable female whose womb-dominated physiology made her especially liable to mental illness or hysteria, and suggests a clear difference between these and the earliest certificates where this is conspicuous by its absence. The age profile of women admitted to the Retreat may also be relevant here since between the ages of 25 and 44 more women (46 per cent) than men (42 per cent) were admitted.

The medical profile of the Retreat's women patients given by computation suggests some interesting differences from those of men and sheds further light on the stereotypes of the female mental patient. In medical diagnoses the main gender differentiation was in the relative proportion of those stated to be suffering from melancholia. In the period before 1843, when diagnostic records were kept systematically, 36 per cent of women, but only 28 per cent of men, were perceived as melancholics. This evidence may qualify the view of woman as rebellious victim, replacing it by an interpretation that gives greater weight to the hidden costs of outward conformity to social constraints. Only one or two cases of moral insanity among the Retreat's female patients give any credence to a view of psychiatric labelling of social deviants; such cases were the exception rather than the norm. But such speculation, though fascinating, raises as many questions as it solves and, in any case, goes beyond the scope of this paper.

Data from the Retreat on recovery rates, duration of stay, and the marital status of female patients largely undercuts the third image concerning the indefinite detention of married women within the asylum. Women had a better chance of recovery; from 1796 to 1910, 39.4 per cent of them were said to have recovered compared to 35.9 per cent of men. And throughout the period single women outnumbered the married at York; in the early years 60 per cent were unmarried and 27 per cent were married, and a century later 56 per cent were single and 36 per cent were married. This growth in the proportion of married women was associated with a declining recruitment of women Quakers — the Society of Friends was notable for the high proportion of spinsters within it during the Victorian period. Both the single and Quakers had relatively longer periods of treatment, and in each of these sub-groups women predominated numerically at the Retreat. It is therefore predictable to find women patients having rather longer periods of treatment at York than did men; fewer women than men were discharged in under a year (41 per cent compared with 45 per cent), and more were there for 10 years or more (21 per cent compared with 17 per cent). The latter may also be explained by the longevity of women.

We turn now to the third subject of enquiry in this section. Low recovery rates in Victorian asylums worried contemporaries since they suggested that earlier buoyant expectations of the specialist institution in providing a cure for insanity were over-optimistic.[11] There was concern over the alleged 'silting-up' of asylums with ageing, chronic cases and suggested remedies included that of non-medical establishments for the incurable. With the benefit of hindsight this discussion may seem misplaced to us when the earlier data in this paper — and comparable data from other asylums — has indicated short duration of stay for the majority of patients. However, it is important to appreciate that there was a small proportion of long-stay patients whose numbers cumulated so that they formed a high proportion of inmates in the institutions at any one time. This point becomes clear if we turn from an analysis of Retreat admissions to that of patients in the asylum at specified census dates. Selecting our census dates as those when there was a change of superintendent, in 1823, 1841, 1849, 1874 and 1892, we find that a fluctuating proportion of between 59 and 74 per cent of first admissions had been there for over ten years. A related, interesting point revealed about the Retreat by this cross-section analysis was the actual age-structure of patients. Whereas the study of age at first admission had indicated that most were in early adulthood or middle age, the age structure revealed for the census dates indicated that for those in the asylum, a variable but high figure of from 33 to 44 per cent were aged 55 years or more. We might therefore conclude that the Victorians had some cause to be anxious about the cumulation of chronic cases, while appreciating both that these formed only a minority of cases treated, and that much larger numbers of patients were being treated for short periods and being discharged as recovered or relieved from their illnesses.

Some problems in quantifying asylum data

The preceding section of this chapter has suggested some examples where quantitative methods are of considerable utility in researching an asylum's history. Yet it must be acknowledged that computing such medical data — unlike that on more objective topics such as gender, age, weight, height, etc. — poses considerable problems; mental illness was (and is) imperfectly understood, was described in ambiguous ways, and furthermore was treated in 'closed' institutions. This section of the paper focuses on problems arising from the quality of the data available in asylum records for computation: the first example discusses the accuracy of statistics provided in the historical records of an asylum; the second the difficulty of converting ambiguous qualitative information into categories suitable for computation; and the third a related issue of whether like is being compared with like in historical records spanning a long time period.

A major problem in using quantitative methods in a study of the asylum can arise from using statistics provided by contemporaries, which on close scrutiny appear to be more misleading than enlightening. After the Lunatics Act of 1845 mental institutions were charged with recording in medical journals their use of seclusion and of mechanical restraint. This record might appear to provide reliable data on a central issue in the mid-Victorian asylum's administration: the practical progress made in implementing the ideals of the non-restraint movement. Further examination of the evidence indicated that a medical officer's definition of what constituted seclusion might differ from those of the Lunacy Commissioners who were responsible for checking the accuracy of these medical records in brief, twice-yearly visits to the asylum.

The pressures that created this divergence are instructive: in the competitive world of asylumdom each establishment attempted to publish in its annual report statistics that were favourable to a progressive image. In these circumstances there was an obvious temptation to construct an impressive record and to minimise any past resort to seclusion or mechanical resort through selective recording. One way to do so was to minute as seclusion cases only those instances in which a patient was sent to a strong room and to turn a blind eye to those more numerous occasions — apparent from the case books — when a patient was secluded informally, for a short period, in their own room in order to regain 'quietness'. The Lunacy Commissioners commented in 1864 that:

> We found a lady locked into her sitting room, which we were
> given to understand had been the case for some hours daily
> during the last few weeks. The reasons given were satisfac-
> tory, but the fact of such seclusion should be entered, as
> such, in the journal.[12]

Such reprimands apparently made little impression and in 1886 a
similar situation was recorded in that the commissioners remarked
that 'if a patient was in bed and likely to leave his room an atten-
dant at the door would prevent his doing so'.[13]

Leaving aside the under-recording that this testimony suggests
happened there was the related issue of what the cases that were
recorded actually meant. Dr Pierce revealed in 1893 that effectively the figures were merely the proverbial 'tip of the iceberg'
since nine minuted cases of seclusion meant that nine patients had
been secluded on 54 occasions for a total period of 335 hours. It
might be assumed that records of the use of mechanical restraint
would be more straightforward and the statistics more accurate
but in fact what constituted restraint was blurred at the edges. For
example, the Lunacy Commissioners noted in 1868 that:

> There is no record of any instances of restraint. It appears
> however that one of the male patients and also a young lady,
> sometimes wear a pair of muffle gloves, which do not confine
> the arms. This fact has hitherto not been reported in the
> medical journal . . .[14]

The superintendent promised that more accurate recording would
be made in the future. However, there were usually means of
circumventing this — either by accident or design. For instance,
these case notes on a suicidally inclined female patient in 1889
recorded that she:

> has injured her throat so much by constantly nipping it with
> her fingers that a dress has been made for her with the
> sleeves sewn to the side and the sleeves at the wrist stitched
> together so as to prevent her from getting at her throat.[15]

In practice this patient was being mechanically restrained but the
form of restraint meant that no record of it needed to be kept.

A second basic difficulty can arise from the ambiguous character of information given in asylum archives and lead to questions of feasibility — or indeed desirability — in using this as the basis for defined categories in computation. A good example is given by the alleged causes of mental disorder in patients' admission certificates. But doubts raised in the historian's mind as to the accuracy of such descriptions were seldom experienced in those of contemporaries. Neat summaries of alleged causes of mental disorder were an obligatory element in any self-respecting Victorian asylum's annual reports, and were also published with confidence by the Commissioners in Lunacy. They divided causation into moral and physical factors. Moral included domestic causes, mental overwork or anxiety, love, fright or shock, religious excitement and adverse business circumstances. Physical factors embraced such diverse elements as physical illness, alcoholism, senility, pregnancy, heredity, change of life, sunstroke, accident and illness. Those who have analysed asylum admissions registers and certificates have added a third mixed category of patients who were given both moral and physical causes for their illness.[16] This mixed category is perhaps the most revealing one since it was designed to fit the frequent miscellany of disparate events and characteristics juxtaposed in the historical record by relatives, friends or doctors in an anxious attempt to make sense of the inexplicable — the onset of mental illness. To facilitate comparisons between the Retreat and other asylums this simple tripartite classification was also adopted in coding Retreat data for the computer.

Let us look at the kind of data that would form the input in such a tripartite categorisation, taking for this purpose entries from the early years of the Retreat's admissions registers. The moral category included entries such as: 'The loss of a son and other afflictions'; 'Over much study'; 'Embarrassment in his affairs'; 'Overstrained nerves particularly on religious subjects'. The physical category included: 'The rickets when an infant impaired her intellect. (Family Comp[lain]t)'; 'The first attack attributed to a profuse use of mercury to a tumour on the nose'; 'A violent blow upon the head by a fall down stairs'; and 'Intemperance'. The mixed category embraced such problematic entries as: 'Enthusiasm in politics and indulgence in liquor added to an hereditary disposition'; 'Family disorder. Perverted education, and an only child much indulged. Cong[enital] peculiarity'; 'Always very irritable. Hereditary? (partly). Disappointed love'; and 'Family complaint. Vanity flattered by success in life. "Fever" 12 years before. [And a later insertion] Masturbation'.[17]

The results of analysing this kind of data for the Retreat's first admissions suggests that in alleged causes of illness mixed factors became less common, physical ones fluctuated in importance, while moral causes assumed increasing weight. In comparison with two pauper asylums where a smaller sample had been analysed by L.J. Ray,[18] the moral factor was given greater significance for the Retreat's admissions. This was perhaps predictable in view of its predominantly middle-class clientele since it was feasible to construct fuller case histories for them. It was also possible to discover through cross-tabulations that, for example, the recovery rate was lower and the death rate higher for the physical cases than the mixed or moral ones. However, although an elaborate hypothesis has been created on the basis of data such as this in another asylum,[19] the quality of these data should make us pause before we accept it uncritically.

Some therapists were themselves either puzzled or sceptical about the significance of alleged causes of mental illness. That the Retreat's therapists were not themselves clear whether they were recording the causation or characteristics of mental illness was suggested by entries such as: 'Hereditary Partly. Religious enthusiasm cause or first symptom'. And they may not have been too confident about the value of an entry such as this example on the supposed origins of imbecility in a patient: 'Not known to be hereditary Lightening [sic]'.[20] Doubts as to the meaning of such data are confirmed when an intelligent contemporary, Frederick Needham (then Superintendent of the York Asylum, who was later a Commissioner in Lunacy and was knighted for his services to psychiatry) poured scorn on the value of his own asylum's statistics on causation, and particularly on the distinction made between predisposing and exciting causes.

> The causes of Insanity, as so described in the 'statement' are, in the majority of instances, utterly unreliable and fictitious; moral influences frequently producing physical infirmities which unjustly receive the credit of originating the mental disorder, and *vice versa*; while the inexactness of observation of a vast proportion of persons unfits them for the appreciation of all but the most obvious and unmistakeable evidences of connection between the causes and the effect, in cases where the former is frequently

complex, and the latter, in its commencement, undefined, and not easily appreciable.[21]

May we therefore conclude that any quantification of the causation of mental illness in the past is an example of 'garbage in and garbage out'? My own view is that there is some historical value and interest in attempting to analyse such data. This resides not so much in supplying accurate information on causation as in throwing light on broad changes in *mentalité* and attempting to gain an insight into the general evolution of contemporaries' views on mental illness. Looked at from this perspective, however, premature 'collapsing' of the data into only three broad categories substantially defeats the objective. To test this proposition it seemed worthwhile to take a smaller, more manageable data set to analyse it in more detail. This was done for patients admitted under Jepson (the first superintendent, 1796–1823), and then for Baker (the latest superintendent, 1874–92, for whom the medical records were reasonably complete). All the specifics given in the alleged causation of mental illness by relatives and doctors were categorised. However, the complexities of the documentation with its changing nuances of meaning effectively 'exploded' my computer coding scheme and led to the analysis being done by more traditional methods. The results suggested some fascinating changes between the two eras. Some reflected more general social changes as in a growing readiness to perceive causation in physical terms; this may be a response both to advances in medical science and to alienists' insistence on the organic basis of mental 'disease'. Other changes may be more specific to the Retreat itself; the decline in the 'hereditary' factor (despite an increasing stress on this in medical literature), probably reflected the shrinking proportion of Quaker patients, as did the lessening importance ascribed to defective education or to ill-regulated conduct. Given the difficulties inherent in these data it is not suggested that any precision can be achieved but rather that this may be one way in which quantitative methods might elucidate a hidden area: broad changes in society's past attitudes to, and perception of, mental illness could be more clearly illuminated.

We now turn to our third problem of whether 'like is being compared with like' and illustrate it with the vexed subject of the outcome attributed by doctors to their patients' treatment. The table summarises the results of their verdicts on the Retreat's first admissions. Of five outcomes only the meaning of 'remain' in the asylum and 'death' are unequivocal. That of 'not improved' is reasonably straightforward since it referred to patients whose treatment was ended very prematurely, as in the case of escaped patients or those removed to a pauper asylum because of financial pressures. The remaining categories of 'relieved' (alternatively 'improved'), and 'recovered' pose real problems of interpretation and thus of comparability. Contemporaries were reluctant to define what was meant by these terms. Indeed, the York Asylum was sufficiently honest to preface its statistical tables of outcomes, for a time, with the statement: 'Recovered, Relieved, not Improved. The Committee has carefully considered these terms and are unable to suggest any definitions which will be universally acceptable. They feel that they must be left to individual interpretation.'[22] Despite this rare disclaimer, those working in the field of mental illness were apparently sufficiently confident of their definitions to compile comparative tables of recovery rates in different asylums.

Some of those at the Retreat attempted to specify what was meant by these terms although their definitions varied. Samuel Tuke — presumably on Jepson's advice — spoke of recovery as 'where the patient is fully competent to fulfil his common duties or is restored to the state he was in previously to the attack'. Dr Thurnam later merely rephrased this in 1845 but Dr Pierce qualified it in 1910 by admitting that 'in many [recovered] cases there remains an instability, a latent tendency to mental disorder, although at the moment [of discharge] no sign of insanity can be discovered'.[23] Was Pierce's greater caution merely a verbal acknowledgement of what was increasingly apparent as the years went by, that a proportion of 'recovered' patients were later re-admitted to the asylum? Or was his actual definition more stringent, and hence his practice in recognising patients as having recovered, more restrictive? Clearly, this point has major implications for any interpretation since computation showed a declining recovery rate from 45.0 per cent under Jepson — superintendent from 1796 to 1823 — to 32.7 per cent under Baker — superintendent from 1874 to 1892. (Deficiencies in data as a result of missing casebooks means that little reliance can be placed on the relative proportion of different kinds of discharge under Baker's successor, Dr Pierce.) Only if it is obvious that there was a constant application of the term 'recovered' is it legitimate to consider possible interpretations for the declining recovery rate, for example, in an evolving emphasis in treatment from moral to

Table 7.1: *Outcome of treatment of first admissions under different superintendents, 1796–1892*

Outcome	Jepson (1796–1823)	Allis (1823–41)	Thurman (1841–49)	Kitching (1849–74)	Baker (1874–92)
Recovery (%)	45.0	44.7	38.4	35.7	32.7
Improved or relieved (%)	11.9	13.5	13.6	16.6	24.0
Not improved (%)	4.2	10.2	10.4	5.5	13.0
Died (%)	38.9	31.6	37.6	41.2	27.7
Remained in 1910 (%)	—	—	—	1.0	2.6
N	260	215	125	308	346
Outcome unknown (%)	—	3	4	26	94

medical, or an altered composition of patient intake.

In this context it is relevant to relate the proportion of patients said to have 'recovered' to those stated to have been merely 'relieved' or 'improved', because perceptions of the boundary between the two states may have altered and thus affected the outcome. Patients in the second category, as we have seen earlier, were usually those who left the asylum on the insistence of friends and before therapists were completely confident that their convalescent state had ended. Therapists' definitions of this state appear to be reasonably consistent: Thurnam suggested that while they no longer required institutional treatment they 'still required the particular care of their friends'; while Pierce stated that the relieved 'still possessed some signs of mental peculiarity'.[24]

Between the time of Jepson and Baker there was a rising proportion of first admissions — from 11.9 to 24.0 per cent — who left the Retreat as 'relieved', and a declining proportion of those who left 'recovered' (see Table 7.1). However, when patients in these two categories of relieved and recovered are taken together they formed a more stable proportion — 56.9 per cent in Jepson's time and 56.7 per cent under Baker. It is possible to interpret this as meaning that the medical criteria for assessing the outcome changed and that there was a flexible boundary between recovered and relieved. Alternatively, non-medical pressures may have been influential in affecting patients' duration of stay. As was suggested earlier the increasing numbers of patients paying economic fees may have led to premature withdrawals of patients and hence to a rise in the proportion of those 'relieved' and a decline in those designated as 'recovered'. It is obvious from this discussion that no easy conclusions are possible in this elusive and ambiguous field, where quantitative methods tend only to expose more clearly the underlying fundamental issues of evaluation and inter-pretation.

The qualitative and the quantitative

There is considerable potential for employing quantitative methods in medical history and to some extent these can be used for investigating the past character and record of psychiatric institutions and their inmates. Quantification facilitates accurate comparisons over time from which to construct a dynamic profile of an institution that challenges the static and over-simplistic portrayals of much ideological writing on the asylum. Com-parisons with other mental institutions are also made much more precise, and hence more useful, if quantification is utilised.

The computation that it is profitable to use in research on the asylum would appear to be more limited than in some other medical fields, if this case study of the Retreat is at all represen-tative of the problems likely to be encountered. Such methods are particularly useful when there are standardised data that are easy to count or code for the computer but, when the information is more fluid or complex, the historian needs to understand its nature very thoroughly indeed before computation is attempted. As the preceding discussion has illustrated, to be able to judge competently whether consistency can be achieved in coding, or whether categories chosen for analysis adequately reflect the nature of the evidence, presents difficulties in dealing with unstan-dardised documentation. Steering a middle way — between the charybdis of prematurely collapsing the data by choosing too few categories for analysis and the scylla of an over-complex analysis that hardly simplifies the original data set — requires considerable foresight and judgement. There are also thorny decisions to be made on whether the time taken to prepare data for computer analysis is likely to be justified by the results: a good example of this would be the use of cluster analysis. The idea of analysing medical case records to detect patterns of language at first seems to be an attractive one. It was rejected in this study of the Retreat because it was thought that there was a low probability of a useful result from what would be a very time-consuming operation.

It will have been apparent that in this study of the Retreat the computer has been used to handle a large data set — large at any rate by the standards of a traditional historian, hitherto working exclusively with a pocket calculator. But the computations performed on this data set have been extremely simple cross-tabulations and frequency distributions. This has yielded some fruitful insights that could not otherwise have been obtained, but it has not exploited the computer's potential. It seems appropriate to end this paper by considering whether more might have been done with the data once they had been stored on the computer. An obvious possibility would have been some form of regression but it appeared that the limitations of much of the data effectively precluded this. For the reasons already discussed the two most interesting medical variables — the causes of mental illness and the outcomes of treatment — were far too uncertain in character to justify their use as elements in a regression analysis. Regression coefficients would give an unwarranted degree of precision to imprecise information. This problem is inherent in the subject since the causation, categorisation, and evaluation of successful treatment of mental illness was, and is, still imperfectly understood. Indeed, it is salutary to discover that the statistical information available on modern psychiatric institutions[25] is a good deal more limited than that on the asylums of the past.

Examining the relationship between the use of the computer and more traditional methods of the historian in researching the history of the asylum raises some interesting issues. At one extreme some topics lend themselves easily to quantification (e.g. the social background and characteristics of patients, certain aspects of the medical record as in the duration of treatment or the number of readmissions). At the other extreme are subjects not easily amenable to quantification (e.g. the evaluation of therapists' characters, or attempts to reconstruct patients' subjective experiences). Within these two 'frontier' areas is a spacious country where both quantitative and qualitative perspectives are useful (e.g. the interpretation of standards in patient care or the evolution of moral treatment into moral management). In many instances these two methodologies provide complementary insights that synthesise into a harmonious interpretation. Yet there are occasions when the two conflict. An example in this study of the Retreat was when quantitative sources on the incidence of and expenditure on drugs contradicted Samuel Tuke's view that medication was minimal in the early years of the asylum. In principle this disagreement is no different from any other conflict of evidence; when the historian encounters this she has to appraise each of the sources carefully in terms of context, accuracy, bias, completeness, etc. Provided that the calibre of the quantitative evidence survives such an examination it would seem in general that it is preferable to the qualitative. And indeed in this instance substantial quantitative data were accepted, rather than the opinion of an individual who lived and worked outside the asylum. There is yet a third predicament when even more difficult problems of evaluation arise because a dialectical process has been set up through divergent lines of interpretation suggested by different methodologies. An illustration would be that of standards of patient care in the era of moral management when quantitative indicators (on such topics as attendant-patient ratios or cases of restraint and seclusion) might indicate improvement, while qualitative evidence from medical case notes (in the use of repressive language or descriptions of violence between attendants and patients) might suggest deterioration. These divergent perspectives suggest the complexities of the issues involved: progress in some areas could coexist with — or even result in — retrograde developments in other aspects of patients' lives. There are no standard procedures or easy answers to deal with this.

Whether the Retreat is seen to retain the essential character of refuge, the 'retired habitation' its founders intended, or whether it developed into a more repressive institution of confinement, is ultimately a matter for the evaluative judgement of the historian in the light of all the available evidence — both quantitative and qualitative. But the asylum is not an easy subject for historical research, and to envisage that increasingly sophisticated methodologies will penetrate all the dark and problematic area within it, is to be over optimistic.

Notes

1. In this context I am more than usually grateful for the numerate assistance given by Charles Feinstein, and also for help in computation by Eileen Sutcliffe.

2. J. Conolly, *Treatment of the Insane without Mechanical Restraint,* (reprinted London, 1973), 17.

3. For example, K. Doerner, *Madmen and the Bourgeoisie. A Social*

History of Insanity and Psychiatry (Oxford, 1981); M. Foucault, *Madness and Civilization. A History of Insanity in the Age of Reason* (London, 1971); A.T. Scull, *Museums of Madness. The Social Organization of Insanity in Nineteenth-Century England* (London, 1979).

4. The Retreat's records are deposited in the Borthwick Institute of Historical Research, York: K/1/1–20 Admissions certificates; J/1/1–2 Admissions Registers; K/2/1–17 Medical case books; J/2 Patients' Survey.

5. *Madness, Morality and Medicine. A Study of the York Retreat, 1796–1910* (Cambridge, 1985); 'The changing profile of a nineteenth-century asylum: the York Retreat', *Psychological Medicine, 14* (1984).

6. Data for the private houses of Hook Norton and Witney are included in W.L. Parry-Jones, *The Trade in Lunacy. A Study of Private Madhouses in the Eighteenth and Nineteenth Centuries* (London, 1972); that for St Thomas's Hospital for Lunatics, later the Asylum for the Four Western Counties in N. Hervey, *Bowhill House* (University of Exeter, 1980); some for Brookwood County Asylum and Lancaster Asylum in L.J. Ray, 'Models of Madness in Victorian Asylum practice', *Arch. Europ. Sociol., XXII* (1981).

7. For the purposes of this analysis Jepson's tenure of office has been extended backwards from the date of his appointment in 1797 to the opening of the asylum in 1796, while Pierce's tenure has been 'ended' in 1910. Thurnam's tenure has been extended backwards to 1841, the date of Allis's resignation.

8. This occupational classification was taken from E. Isichei, *Victorian Quakers* (Oxford, 1970) as a means of comparing the occupational background of Retreat patients with those in the Society of Friends analysed there.

9. See E. Showalter, 'Victorian Women and Insanity', in A. Scull (ed.), *Madness, Mad-Doctors and Madmen. The Social History of Psychiatry in the Victorian Era* (London, 1981), 313–38.

10. For these theories at their most highly developed see H. Maudsley, *The Pathology of Mind,* 2nd edn (London, 1895); T.S. Clouston, *Clinical Lectures on Mental Diseases,* 4th edn (London, 1896); C. Mercier, *A Textbook of Insanity* (London, 1902). See also my forthcoming paper on the link between gynaecological and psychiatric literature, 'Women's biological straitjacket' in S. Mendus and J. Rendall (eds.), *Images of Women: The Victorian Legacy* (in press, 1987).

11. Scull, *Museums of Madness,* 190, 192.

12. Borthwick Institute, G/1/1, Reports of Visiting Commissioners in Lunacy, 27 January 1864.

13. G/1/1, 4 November 1886.

14. G/1/1, 27 November 1864.

15. Borthwick Institute, K/2/16, Medical case book, case 1662, observation 15 November 1889.

16. Ray 'Models of Madness', 264.

17. Borthwick Institute, J/1/1 Admissions register, cases 60, 74, 92, 106, 108, 155, 173, 185, 202, 400, 442.

18. Ray 'Models of Madness'.

19. Ray 'Models of Madness'.

20. Borthwick Institute, J/1/1, cases 186, 656.

21. Bootham Park Hospital, *Report of York Lunatic Asylum* (1869), 11.

22. *Report of York Lunatic Asylum* (1915).

23. S. Tuke, *Description of the Retreat*, 2nd edn (London, 1964), 216; J. Thurnam, *Statistics of Insanity* (London, 1845), 29; Retreat *Report* (1910).

24. Thurnam, *Statistics,* 30; Retreat *Report* (1904).

25. *The Facilities and Services of Mental Illness and Mental Handicap Hospitals in England* (DHSS Statistical and Research Report Series 21, 1980).

8

Hospital History : New Sources and Methods

Guenter B. Risse

Most histories of hospitals have hitherto been simple narratives narrowly focused on a particular institution, frequently commissioned to celebrate special anniversaries in their evolution. In such circumstances, these individual accounts take on the character of an official repository of prominent individuals who, as benefactors and healers, held important appointments in the hospital. The stories, sprinkled here and there with anecdotes, usually unfold inside the institutional walls, detached from the contemporary social context that could provide a broader perspective of the events.[1]

Not surprisingly, therefore, such descriptive histories of hospitals fail to probe the actual nature and operations of institutional confinement. Aside from stressing a positivistic view of medical progress, they remain silent about the actual details of institutional management, especially medical therapy. Moreover, the meaning, status and economic benefits provided for medical professionals by the hospital affiliation are seldom explored.

Patients and their ailments also frequently remain in the background, overshadowed by the prominence accorded to healers and benefactors. Indeed, such histories even fail to probe the criteria employed for admitting and discharging individuals from the hospital, as well as the rationales adduced by physicians for planning treatment. Perhaps more importantly, these stories totally ignore issues important for patients that are inherent in the process of hospitalisation: dependence, depersonalisation, and isolation from family networks.

One could actually argue that such historiographic efforts have created a paradox: perused individually, particular hospital histories portray successful developments achieved through the efforts of particular dedicated men and women. However, when viewed collectively from a social and epidemiological point of view, hospitals have been categorised as 'hotbeds of infection' or even 'death traps', only visited by poor people as places of last resort.[2] The former view focuses almost exclusively on the presence of health professionals who made up the hospital staffs and gallantly waged war on disease. The latter, by contrast, assesses the general impact of hospitalisation on society and patients against some ideal but vague common 'good'. The two perspectives, it would appear, cannot be easily reconciled, but how are we to obtain a comprehensive picture of hospital life capable of transcending such common stereotypes?

In calling for a new institutional history of hospitals, I am aware of the need for new sources of information. Thus, the rest of this paper will concentrate on the materials and the knowledge they can provide for such a history. Published statistics or annual reports, official regulations or statutes, and minutes of meetings held by hospital governing boards may be available in many instances. Important additions can be general registers of patients, admission and discharge lists, ward journals, prescription books, and apothecary inventories. Finally, it will be possible in some cases to obtain clinical histories of hospitalised individuals, selectively published in journal articles, physicians' casebooks, or hospital ledgers.

Why are all these sources important? Let me use examples from my recent study concerning the Royal Infirmary of Edinburgh to illustrate them.[3] The annual hospital reports usually provide a complete list of current contributors, thus revealing their number, geographic location, and social status. At times, one can assess the spectrum of donors and thus uncover the network of local leadership concerned with philanthropic matters and institutional governance. At Edinburgh, members of the nobility, professionals, prominent merchants, and even some local ship captains provided financial assistance.[4] Moreover, money obtained from subscriptions reveals the relative importance of this income in relation to other, perhaps more stable, sources of hospital revenue. At Edinburgh, for example, a subscription system appeared only late, during the economic difficulties brought on by Britain's war with France. By 1800, these contributions barely amounted to 6 per cent of the total income, compared with the 20 per cent obtained from the sale of student tickets, 15 per cent for the care of sick seamen from the Royal Navy, and 10 per cent received as rent from a property in Jamaica.[5]

When available, such financial records can be quite revealing. In the case of the Edinburgh Infirmary, one can find, on a yearly basis, a number of treasurer's accounts that itemised sources of both income and expense. This allows historians to not only assess the overall fate of a hospital budget, but the relative position of such items as building maintenance and repair, fuel bills in the form of coal and candles, salaries, food and laundry costs, etc. One puzzling development, which may have been unique for Edinburgh, was the steady decrease of expenditures for drugs in spite of rapidly growing admission rates. Whether the decline reflects changing patterns of drug utilisation by physicians, both in number and dosages, or is merely an artefact of greater institutional self-sufficiency — the Infirmary had access to a 'physic garden' and could therefore grow some of its own medicinal herbs — needs further study.

Minutes of the meetings held by a hospital's board of governors or managers usually disclose important information regarding professional policy, financial matters, staff appointments, and new regulations. From time to time, these documents allow glimpses of personality conflicts, professional tensions (at Edinburgh the struggle between attending physicians and surgeons), disruptive behaviour by the staff (medical clerks and nurses), and sustained efforts to balance budgetary matters (greater fundraising efforts). Events such as written complaints, official reprimands, periodic inspections, hiring and firing of personnel, and legal actions greatly help to flesh out the institutional affairs.[6]

In turn, hospital statistics published in separate annual reports or medical journals — during the 18th century the Edinburgh Infirmary published its figures for several decades in *Scots Magazine* — are very revealing. Not only do they provide total admission and discharge figures, but often record the occupancy rate as of January 1, or give various categories of patients' discharge from the institution. In the case of the Edinburgh Infirmary, the managers for several years also characterised the patients as 'ordinary' (charitable, non-paying) or 'supernumerary' (paying a daily fee), and also listed separately soldiers, servants, and seamen.[7]

Of even greater importance, when available, are general registers of patients. This source provides a list of all the admitted patients, their destination within the hospital, diagnoses, as well as dates of admission and discharge, and the category of such a discharge. Through an examination of patients' first names, researchers can easily determine the sex distribution among those individuals who came to the institution. Their in-house destination often provides clues about their occupation, as in the case of the Edinburgh Infirmary, where large numbers of patients went into wards specifically reserved for servants, soldiers, and seamen.[8]

Admission and discharge dates, in turn, are valuable for computing the length of hospitalisation, and establish seasonal patterns for the acceptance of persons suffering from ailments such as fevers, respiratory ailments, rheumatism, and malaria. At the Edinburgh Infirmary, a gradual shortening of the period of hospitalisation for many patients between 1770 and 1800 allowed for a faster turnover in the wards and an increased number of annual admissions.

Moreover, discharge categories usually listed in hospital registers permit some judgments regarding the overall cure and mortality rate, the number of patients considered 'relieved', those who were dismissed 'by desire', or for 'irregularities'. Equally important are the categories 'improper' and 'incurable', since they provide us with clues about the perceived limits of contemporary medicine.

Finally, general hospital registers also contain a large number of diagnostic labels, often merely repeating the principal complaint: fever, cough, bruise, sore leg, itch, and pain.[9] The task of understanding the nature of all such ailments recorded in a register of patients without violating their original meaning is not easy. Researchers are all too prone to replace old labels with modern medical terms, thereby distorting and at times seriously misinterpreting the data. Therefore, I would like to offer a model that preserves older categories — in this case, 18th century classifications — while at the same time making sense of them in terms of modern knowledge. In the case of the Edinburgh Infirmary, the original diagnoses were first separated into a medical and another surgical group by checking the destination of each patient after admission as recorded in the register. Next, both of these groups were subdivided into a number of broad categories that reflected the original character of the disease as perceived by 18th century physicians. Thus, for example, lues venerea was placed under the category of genito-urinary diseases, together with 'gravel', 'diabetes', and 'amenorrhoea'. 'Pectoral complaint', in turn, was listed as a respiratory disease with 'dyspnoea', 'asthma', 'cough', and 'phthisis'.

In this fashion, all original diagnostic labels taken from the General Register of Patients of the Edinburgh Infirmary between 1770 and 1800 were arranged under the following categories:

Medical diseases (76.1 per cent)   *Surgical diseases* (20.2 per cent)

(a) genito-urinary   (a) infectious
(b) infectious   (b) trauma
(c) respiratory   (c) tumours
(d) digestive   (d) surgical procedures
(e) musculo-skeletal   (e) miscellaneous
(f) neurological-mental
(g) skin
(h) circulatory
(i) eye problems
(j) miscellaneous

A complete list of all the old diagnoses arranged under the new categories is appended (see Table 8.1 and 8.2). Although this method allowed most 18th-century labels to be included, a small miscellaneous category was added for both medical and surgical conditions with ambiguous designations such as 'debility', 'convalescence', and 'anomalous complaint'.[10]

To establish the relative frequency of diagnoses made at the hospital, one can randomise the data provided in many general registers of patients. For the Edinburgh Infirmary, entries were obtained from the General Register of Patients for the years 1770, 1775, 1780, 1785, 1790, 1795 and 1800. Using the patients' registrations inscribed on every fourth folio, a random sample of 3,047 diagnoses was created, and the various labels distributed among the previously established medical and surgical categories.[11]

Not surprisingly, the genito-urinary category came out on top simply because large numbers of soldiers and seamen suffering from venereal diseases were routinely admitted to the Infirmary in accordance with arrangements approved by both the hospital authorities and the Commander-in-Chief of the Armed Forces. The distribution among the sexes showed that more than two-thirds of the patients with these diseases were men (Table 8.3).

It should be clear, however, that this hospital morbidity is by no means representative of the diseases that afflicted the local population. Social criteria of eligibility ('the deserving poor'), contractual obligations (servants, soldiers and seamen), and only moderately sick people 'proper' for hospital treatment (most

Table 8.1: Royal Infirmary of Edinburgh General Register of Patients 1770–1800. Medical disease categories.

1. *Genito-urinary diseases*

Amenorrhoea	Phymosis	Diabetes	Nephritis
Chlorosis	Sibbens	Bladder disease	Painful bladder
Gonorrhoea	Swollen testicles	Dysuria	Stone
Leucorrhoea	Syphilis	Enuresis	Urinary
Lues venerea	Anuria	Gravel	complaint
Menorrhagia	Calculus	Ischuria	

2. *Infectious diseases*

Ague or intermittent fever	Pertussis or whooping cough
Fever	Scarlatina or scarlet fever
Hectic fever	Smallpox
Measles	Tabes
Mumps	Typhus fever

3. *Respiratory ailments*

Angina	Cough	Inflammed breast	Pneumonia
Asthma	Catarrh	Pectoral complaint	Phthisis
Breast complaint	Cynanche	Pleuresy	Sore throat
Breast pain	Dyspnoea	Pain (in) breast	
Cold	Haemoptysis	Pain (in) side	

4. *Diseases of the digestive system*

Bilious complaint	Crampish pains	Dyspepsia	Jaundice
Bowel complaint	Costiveness	Stomach complaint	Icterus
Cholera	Diseased liver	Enteritis	Typanites
Colic or spasm	Diarrhoea	Hepatitis	Vomiting
Colica pictonum	Dysentery	Ileus	Worms

5. *Musculo-skeletal disorders*

Atrophy	Ischias	Spasm of breast
Back pain	Lumbago	Stiff arm and joint
Diseased ankle, arm,	Pain (in) arm, knee, leg	Strained thigh
finger, hip, knee, leg	Rheumatism	Swollen wrist
or toe	Rickets	Tetanus
	Sciatica	Weak arm

6. *Neurological-mental diseases*

Atrophy	Head complaint	Hypochondriasis
Chorea	Hemiplegia	Hysteria
Concussion	Lethargy	Mania
Deafness	Paralysis or palsy	Melancholy
Epilepsy	Phrenitis	Nostalgia
Headaches	Vertigo	Senility

7. *Diseases of the skin*

Chilblain	Lepra
Eruption	Psora or itch
Erysipelas or the rose	Scurvy
Herpes	Scorbutic eruption
Impetigo	Tinea or white head

Table 8.1: continued.

8. *Circulatory disorders*

Aneurysm	Dropsy	Hydrothorax
Anasarca	Haemorrhoids	Plethora
Ascites	Hydrocephalus	Congestion

9. *Eye problems*

Amaurosis	Opacity (of) cornea
Caligo	Ophthalmia

10. *Miscellaneous medical conditions*

Anomalous complaint	Feigned complaints
Convalescence	Inoculation (smallpox)
Debility	Pain

Table 8.2: Royal Infirmary of Edinburgh General Register of Patients 1770–1800. Surgical disease categories.

1. *Surgical infections*

Abscesses	Sores	Suppurations	Phlegmons
Bone caries	Sore (on) leg	Swellings	Ulcers
Fistulas	Sore (on) foot	White swellings	Ulcer (on) leg

2. *Traumatic conditions*

Accident	Dog bite	Mortification of feet
Bruise or contusion	Fracture (of) leg, arm	Sprain (of) ankle
Burn	finger, rib, skull,	hand, thigh, wrist
Cut (on) leg, head, knee	thigh, eye, foot, leg	Wound
Discolouration (of) ankle,	Luxation	Wound or hurt foot,
arm, leg, spine, thigh		head, scalp, throat

3. *Tumors and cancers*

Cancer (of) breast,	Scrophula	Steatoma
lip	Schirrhous tumour	Tumour (of) back,
Exostosis	Schirrhous testicle,	cheek, jaw, lip, knee,
Polyp	tonsil, uterus	testicle, thigh

4. *Surgical procedures*

Amputation	Lithotomy
Castration	Trephined skull

5. *Miscellaneous surgical conditions*

Cataract	Hydrocele	Stricture of urethra
Harelip	Imperforated rectum	Umbilical hernia
Hernia	Odontalgia	

---

*Table 8.3: Royal Infirmary of Edinburgh General Register of Patients,
1770–1800. Sex differential for the diagnostic categories.*

Category	Male	Female
	(Percentage)	
Medical diseases	60.5	39.1
Genito-urinary	71.9	28.0
Infectious	53.6	46.1
Respiratory	60.6	39.3
Digestive	51.9	47.5
Musculo-skeletal	62.6	37.3
Neurol-mental	40.6	58.6
Skin	60.9	35.9
Miscellaneous	59.7	40.2
Surgical diseases	63.9	36.0
Infectious	61.3	38.6
Trauma	71.0	28.9
Tumours	60.0	40.0
Surgical procedures	63.1	36.8
Miscellaneous	72.0	28.0
Unknown	63.6	35.4

smallpox patients were unacceptable) created effective barriers. Unfortunately, such a filter does not allow inferences regarding the epidemiology in the so-called 'catchment' area surrounding the hospital.[12]

Further information delivered from patients' registers deals with the in-house distribution of those who were hospitalised. Of interest was the composition of a special teaching ward in the Edinburgh Infirmary under the direction of professors teaching at the local Medical School. Virtually all cases were of a medical nature. Also noteworthy was the absence in the servant's ward of cases diagnosed as suffering from venereal diseases, quite prevalent in the soldier's ward. Servants suffered instead more from fevers and skin eruptions, two highly visible health problems that seemingly brought them to the attention of their masters (Table 8.4).

Using the registration data for specific years, one can chart a distribution of the various disease categories over time and also investigate the possibility that admitting physicians modified their perceptions and criteria concerning certain diagnoses, perhaps in response to new medical knowledge or the adoption of other classification systems. At the Edinburgh Infirmary, for example,

Table 8.4: Royal Infirmary of Edinburgh General Register of Patients, 1770–1800. Diagnostic categories and their distribution in the hospital wards (percentages).

	Medical	Surgical	Teaching	Soldiers	Servants	Seamen
Medical diseases	49.4	2.8	10.9	21.4	12.6	2.4
Genito-urinary	39.6	2.5	5.2	47.4	2.8	1.5
Infectious	46.1	0.4	12.0	16.0	21.6	3.7
Respiratory	48.7	1.5	12.5	16.5	16.5	3.7
Digestive	66.1	0.9	12.7	3.4	15.2	0.9
Musculo-skeletal	59.5	7.0	10.8	6.6	13.2	2.7
Neurol-mental	62.4	0.7	15.0	6.7	12.7	2.2
Skin	49.2	5.4	7.8	15.6	18.7	3.1
Miscellaneous	50.9	9.4	23.9	8.1	6.9	0.6
Surgical diseases	13.1	67.7	1.9	11.2	4.7	1.1
Infectious	12.4	66.3	2.4	12.9	5.2	0.5
Trauma	7.2	79.6	1.3	4.6	5.9	1.3
Tumours	33.3	49.3	—	13.3	2.6	—
Surgical procedures	—	100.0	—	—	—	—
Miscellaneous	8.0	48.0	4.0	28.0		12.0
Unknown	40.9	34.5	10.0	9.0	2.7	1.8

the admission of cases of venereal diseases declined significantly between the years 1770–1800,[13] in part because proportionately fewer soldiers entered the hospital, but also because other ailments such as typhus fever, malaria, and rheumatism became more frequent. Noteworthy was the steady rise in traumatic surgical cases, many of them accidents that were inevitable consequences of urbanisation. Trauma cases, in fact, virtually doubled in Edinburgh during the three decades under study (Table 8.5).

Looking at possible seasonal variations in the admission of patients with certain diagnoses, the computer-assisted analysis of our random sample from the General Register of Patients was quite useful. As expected, the most obvious correlations were obtained between respiratory ailments and hospital admissions during the months of December and January. By contrast, so-called 'fevers' were actually more common during the autumn, while cases of 'rheumatism' and 'nervous' problems came in more frequently during the summer.

The ready availability of both admission and discharge dates in general registers makes it possible to calculate the length of hospital stay of patients. In the Edinburgh study, hospitalisation

Table 8.5: Royal Infirmary of Edinburgh General Register of Patients, 1770–1800. Yearly distribution of diagnostic categories (percentage).

	1770	1775	1780	1785	1790	1795	1800	Total average
Medical diseases	82.4	81.3	72.0	81.0	73.6	69.1	71.2	75.8
Genito-urinary	40.3	20.4	26.3	22.8	31.6	29.1	24.6	27.9
Infectious	16.9	21.5	20.3	30.8	17.4	12.6	20.7	20.1
Respiratory	9.4	15.5	11.3	8.4	17.4	16.4	18.8	13.9
Digestive	7.1	8.1	11.3	7.4	11.8	7.8	7.6	8.7
Musculo-skeletal	10.6	13.1	9.6	10.0	9.4	13.0	12.4	11.1
Neurolo-mental	6.3	7.3	5.6	6.1	3.5	6.5	4.7	5.7
Skin	5.1	10.1	5.6	5.6	3.2	5.8	2.5	5.4
Miscellaneous	3.9	3.5	9.6	8.4	5.3	8.5	8.3	6.8
Surgical diseases	13.0	16.8	23.0	18.3	25.0	29.6	17.3	20.4
Infectious	70.0	90.7	67.2	42.0	44.3	50.4	50.0	59.2
Trauma	12.5	6.5	15.0	38.6	29.5	30.4	25.0	22.5
Tumours	12.5	—	7.9	15.9	15.6	14.4	14.4	11.5
Surgical procedures	2.5	1.3	4.4	2.2	4.3	2.4	2.6	2.8
Miscellaneous	2.5	1.3	5.3	1.1	6.0	2.4	7.8	3.8
Unknown	4.5	1.7	4.8	0.6	1.3	1.1	11.3	3.6

periods fluctuated significantly, perhaps because social considerations rather than purely medical criteria played an important role in the decision to discharge patients.[14] Nevertheless, data from the random sample suggest that overall hospitalisation decreased gradually over the three decades, from an average of 43 to 28 days for most conditions, thereby allowing for a greater turnover of patients and increasingly higher admission rates. Venereal diseases and surgically treated infections required an average of six weeks in the hospital while most patients suffering from other medical conditions only remained in the wards for four weeks (Table 8.6).

Finally, general hospital registers often recorded the discharge category assigned to departing patients. In the computer-assisted study of the Edinburgh Infirmary, almost two-thirds of those discharged were judged to be 'cured', a somewhat ambiguous term that variously meant total recovery, apparent convalescence, or simply freedom from the presenting complaints. An alternative category was 'relieved', often implying that the condition was incurable but also signalling symptomatic improvement. Very important for the public image of the hospital was the institutional

Table 8.6: *Royal Infirmary of Edinburgh General Register of Patients,*
1770–1800. Length of hospitalisation.

Disease category	Average stay (days)
Medical	29.1
Genito-urinary diseases	42.3
Infectious diseases	24.7
Respiratory ailments	23.7
Diseases of the digestive system	27.3
Musculo-skeletal disorders	30.2
Neurological-mental diseases	34.2
Diseases of the skin	31.0
Miscellaneous medical conditions	30.4
Surgical	40.0
Surgical infections	42.8
Traumatic conditions	32.5
Tumours and cancers	38.0
Surgical procedures	55.1
Miscellaneous surgical conditions	38.2

mortality rate, deliberately kept low through careful selection of patients and the discharge of moribund inmates. Another useful gauge of the patient's acceptance of hospital treatment was the discharge 'by desire' of those who grew tired and disappointed by the lack of improvement or tried to dodge specific modes of medical treatment such as bloodletting and blistering. In turn, the category 'for irregularities' was reserved for patients who disobeyed medical orders or violated hospital rules. Headings such as 'incurable', 'improper', and 'by advice' were usually reserved for individuals whose conditions were no longer suitable for hospital treatment, with the latter two categories still suggesting a chance for recovery outside the institution.[15]

Again, studying the data obtained from the Edinburgh Infirmary, discharges labelled 'cured' gradually decreased over the years of the study, especially in the period corresponding to the Napoleonic wars (Table 8.7). Such a shift was due in part to an increase in the admissions of respiratory and circulatory disorders that always exhibited higher mortality indices. Another plausible explanation for these changes at Edinburgh was the serious deterioration of hospital care because of financial difficulties. It most directly compromised the quality of the diet offered to patients as well as affected the overall cleanliness of the institution, especially because of problems with the laundry and water supply.[16]

Table 8.7: Royal Infirmary of Edinburgh General Register of Patients, 1770–1800. Discharge status related to particular years and distinguished by sex.

Year	Cured		Relieved		Dead	
	Male	Female	Male	Female	Male	Female
1770	73.0	76.5	14.5	9.3	2.7	0.7
1775	83.2	85.4	6.6	2.6	3.8	4.6
1780	67.0	69.1	10.3	9.0	4.3	2.3
1785	70.0	71.0	11.0	11.5	5.5	3.6
1790	71.0	69.8	13.6	17.6	2.6	3.1
1795	62.5	71.1	13.5	15.4	5.7	4.9
1800	61.0	57.3	4.5	9.5	6.0	4.4
Total average	69.5	71.6	10.4	10.4	4.4	3.4

The second part of this study about potential sources for the history of hospitals focuses on a rare but rich source of data: individual clinical histories. Certain institutions preserved ward journals and ledgers containing abbreviated or complete patient cases. In the case of Edinburgh, such journals fell prey to the ravages of time or were recycled during periodic paper shortages. Fortunately, however, late-18th-century medical students directly copied a fair number of cases from the official hospital records of the teaching ward and then went on to preserve these casebooks in their private libraries. Now available in several British and American archives, the notebooks provide valuable information about patient care and the progress of individual patients in an 18th-century institutional setting such as the Royal Infirmary of Edinburgh.[17]

Data cited in this portion of the Edinburgh study were extracted from fourteen separate student casebooks containing a total of 808 complete cases from the years 1771 to 1799 (Table 8.8). Each document contains approximately 50–60 clinical histories that often provide the name, age, and occasionally occupation and marital status of the individual patient. Admission dates, statements about the duration of complaints prior to admittance and treatment before hospitalisation are followed by a description of the principal complaints and their relationship to predisposing and precipitating causes. Initial dietary recommendations, drug prescriptions, and physical measures such as fomentations, bathing, or bloodletting are then noted, all written in Latin. Virtually every day progress notes and new therapeutic

Table 8.8: Royal Infirmary of Edinburgh. Student casebooks 1771–1799.

Professor in charge	Date	No. of cases	Location
John Gregory	1771–72	50	Medical Archives, Univ. of Edinburgh
William Cullen	1772–73	52	National Library of Medicine, Washington
William Cullen	1773–74	34	National Library of Medicine, Washington
James Gregory	1779–80	85	Royal College of Physicians, Edinburgh
Francis Home	1780–81	55	Royal College of Physicians, Edinburgh
John Hope	1781	33	University of Edinburgh
James Gregory	1781–82	104	Royal College of Physicians, Edinburgh
James Gregory	1785–86	57	University of Edinburgh
Francis Home	1786–87	52	Edinburgh City Library
Andrew Duncan, Sr.	1795	65	Royal College of Physicians, Edinburgh
James Gregory	1795–96	64	University of Edinburgh, Edinburgh
Thomas C. Hope	1796–97	63	Royal College of Physicians, Edinburgh
Daniel Rutherford	1799	94	Royal College of Physicians, Edinburgh
Total		808	

orders were subsequently appended to the case history until the patient was finally dismissed or transferred to another hospital ward. Date and category of discharge were also recorded. For the 18th century, the wealth of information thus obtained is quite extraordinary.

Before proceeding with the computer-assisted analysis of the Edinburgh casebooks, it should be noted, however, that all 808 patients contained in them were not representative of the Infirmary population as a whole. In most instances, these individuals were admitted to the teaching ward because their complaints sounded 'interesting', the case was 'challenging' as a problem in medical management or the professor in charge of the unit just happened to be lecturing on the disease they suffered from. However, in spite of the double selection process to become a 'proper' hospital and teaching case, every patient history provides very useful and detailed knowledge not readily available elsewhere.

In many ways these data nicely supplement those obtained from patient registers. For the Edinburgh study, the most obvious discrepancies between facts derived from the General Register and the casebooks was the predominance of female patients in the latter. Moreover, the teaching cases were exclusively medical in nature, and their significantly higher mortality rate — double that of the institution at large — reveals a patient population afflicted with more severe and complicated health problems.[18]

What information can be extracted from the individual cases? First, one can determine the average age of the patients; in the case of Edinburgh (28.6 years), with women slightly younger (25.5) than men (32.7). Occupations were seldom included, but their range was extensive, from agricultural workers (farmers, fowlers, millers, and ploughmen) to industrial labourers (lead, glass, and copper-plate workers). Moreover, among the tradesmen were weavers, carters, masons, butchers, painters, and wrights, together with an array of servants (coachmen, footmen, gardeners and waiters). Average ages recorded were for labourers (40), seamen (32), soldiers (25) and servants (22).

Another important measurement made in this study was the duration of the patient's complaints before admission to the hospital, information presumably obtained by the admitting physician during the initial history-taking session. This knowledge served to characterise each ailment as being *acute* (fewer than 10 days of symptoms), *sub-acute* (10–30 days), or *chronic* (over 30 days). Although the intermediary sub-acute category was not employed at that time, 18th-century perceptions of acuteness and chronicity were checked by using a frequent contemporary disease, 'rheumatism', which physicians often labelled either acute or chronic. Not surprisingly, one can find an exact correlation in virtually all cases between the 18th-century and modern criteria, except for some blurring of distinctions between what we now label sub-acute and chronic. By these measurements, all 808 teaching cases from the Edinburgh Infirmary between the years 1771 and 1799 can be characterised as follows:

acute   39.5 per cent
sub-acute   23.6 per cent
chronic   36.8 per cent

If such distributions are in turn related to the patient's age, it becomes clear that younger individuals logically suffered more from acute diseases while older patients were affected by sub-acute and chronic health problems. If the data are analysed by gender, females seem to have been struck more frequently with acute sickness, whereas males tolerated their complaints longer before seeking hospital admission.

Another useful fact derived from clinical histories is the statement regarding medical treatments received prior to hospitalisation. In the sample derived from student casebooks, 47 per cent of the patients admitted to such therapeutic efforts. Duration of the complaints was certainly an important factor in seeking therapy. Only a third of the patients with acute conditions received it, while fully half of those persons with long-standing, chronic complaints requested some remedies. It is interesting to note that, proportionally, younger patients, and females in particular, failed either to solicit or to receive such medical therapy.

The nature and frequency of patient complaints recorded in the clinical histories are summarised in Tables 8.9 and 8.10, the latter arranged by gender. From the data, it appears that female patients admitted to the Edinburgh Infirmary had a slightly higher incidence of symptoms expressed as chills and heat, the result of a greater influx of fever cases. Indeed, professors in charge of the teaching ward often admitted significant numbers of young febrile females to illustrate their extensive lectures on the topic before students.[19]

Clinical histories contained in student casebooks usually

Table 8.9: *Royal Infirmary of Edinburgh. Student casebooks 1771–1799.*
Frequency of symptoms (808 cases)

Symptom	No. of cases (per cent)	
Pain	459	(16.9)
Heat (fever)	232	(8.5)
Cough	204	(7.5)
Swelling	200	(7.3)
Debility	172	(6.3)
Chills	171	(6.3)
Dyspnoea	168	(6.2)

Table 8.10: *Royal Infirmary of Edinburgh. Student casebooks 1771–1799.*
Frequency of symptoms by sex (percentage)

Symptom	Males	Females
Pain	41.8	58.1
Heat (fever)	37.5	62.5
Cough	46.0	53.9
Swelling	50.0	50.0
Debility	45.3	54.6
Chills	39.1	60.8
Dyspnoea	47.0	52.9
Overall percentage of cases	43.1	56.8

presented specific clusters of symptoms. Their presence in these
documents is probably a reflection of age-old symptomatic
associations — almost stereotypical — made by the 18th-century
interviewers who then went on to record their appearance in
patients. In order of frequency among the 808 cases they were:

1. Chills-heat-headaches (febrile illness)
2. Dyspnoea-cough-expectoration (respiratory)
3. Anorexia-nausea-vomiting-indigestion (gastric)
4. Pain-stiffness of joints-swelling (rheumatic)
5. Abdominal cramps-flatulence-constipation or diarrhoea
   (intestinal)
6. Numbness-vertigo-paralysis (neurological)

Table 8.11 analyses the most prominent symptoms and
correlates their presence with frequency of medical treatment

Table 8.11: *Royal Infirmary of Edinburgh. Student casebooks 1771–1799. Treatment of presenting symptoms prior to admission (percentage).*

Symptom	
Pain	50
Heat (fever)	39
Cough	39
Swelling	50
Debility	52
Chills	39
Dyspnoea	39

prior to hospitalisation. Not unexpectedly, the presence of pain prompted patients to seek help in at least half of the cases.

Critical components of the information derived from notebooks were the diagnostic labels attached to each case. Their distribution in the Edinburgh teaching ward differs significantly from that observed in the institution's General Register of Patients.[20] Indeed, the teaching unit accepted a greater number of infectious cases (28 per cent) compared with the hospital at large (15 per cent), while virtually no venereal problems were admitted (2 per cent), hospital (20 per cent). Discrepancies concerning other categories were less noticeable: respiratory diseases, teaching ward 17 per cent, hospital 11 per cent; gastro-intestinal problems, teaching ward 11 per cent, hospital 6 per cent.

Correlations between certain diagnostic labels and age as well as the gender of patients yielded equally interesting conclusions. Females were certainly overrepresented among infectious and skin diseases, while males suffered proportionally more from respiratory, gastro-intestinal and neurological disorders (Table 8.12). When arranged by age, older patients seemed to have been more affected by circulatory and urinary problems while the young had infections (Table 8.13).

For the first time, student casebooks allow a close look at medical treatments individually prescribed for patients in the Edinburgh Infirmary. Most of the contemporary textbooks and even selected reports in medical journals usually deal with the subject of therapeutics in a generalised, prescriptive manner without furnishing precise details or even dosages of the drugs employed. In these hospital cases, however, the reader discovers specific instructions and detailed prescriptions. Moreover notes appear about the effects of such measures, repeated drug

Table 8.12: Royal Infirmary of Edinburgh. Student casebooks 1771–1799. Diagnostic categories and their sex distribution.

Diagnosis	Total cases	Males	Females	Total percentage
Infectious diseases	233	89	144	28.8
Respiratory	139	73	66	17.2
Gastro-intestinal	91	48	43	11.2
Musculo-skeletal	81	34	47	10.0
Neurological	70	43	27	8.6
Circulatory	55	28	27	6.8
Skin	34	8	26	4.2
Gynaecological	30	—	30	3.7
Mental	25	5	20	3.0
Venereal	18	14	4	2.2
Urinary	17	10	7	2.1
Tumours	11	5	6	1.3
Miscellaneous	4	—	4	0.4
Totals	808	357	451	

Table 8.13: Royal Infirmary of Edinburgh. Student casebooks 1771–1799. Average patient age and diagnostic categories.

Diagnosis	Age (years)
Urinary diseases	41.0
Circulatory disorders	38.8
Respiratory diseases	30.5
Tumours	30.5
Gastro-intestinal	30.2
Neurological	30.0
Musculo-skeletal	29.6
Venereal	28.3
Gynaecological	28.0
Skin problems	27.4
Mental	26.0
Infectious	24.3

substitutions, or even fundamental shifts in therapeutic approach taken in response to changes observed in the patient under treatment.

To bring some order to the analysis of hospital therapy, all measures instituted for this purpose were separated into two categories: drugs and physical methods.[21] The former were, in turn, divided into a number of classes in accordance with prevailing 18th-century concepts. Similarly, physical methods such as

Table 8.14: Royal Infirmary of Edinburgh. Student casebooks 1771–1799.
Drug utilisation in hospital practice.

Drug	Prescriptions (%)	
Purgatives	523	(26.2)
Anodynes or pain	326	(16.3)
Emetics	278	(14.0)
Diaphoretics	217	(10.8)
Expectorants	162	(8.1)
Tonics	151	(7.5)
Diuretics	111	(5.5)
Mercurials	87	(4.3)

blistering, bathing, bloodletting, and electricity were considered separately. All cures were related to the previously established disease categories and their relative frequency of utilisation discovered with the help of a computer. More importantly, variations in the use of drugs and physical measures among individual Edinburgh professors were determined by comparing therapeutic measures described in separate student casebooks.

All prescriptions listed in the casebooks were examined and their major drugs identified. The Edinburgh study used eight categories established by contemporary 18th-century practitioners.[22] As Table 8.14 indicates, purgatives lead all other groups represented. When linked with the various disease categories, purgatives appear to have been routinely prescribed in about two-thirds of all cases regardless of the ailment under treatment. The same generic employment can also be found in the use of analgesics and emetics (Table 8.15). More specific indications can be noted in the prescription of diaphoretics (sweat-inducing compounds) in the treatment of rheumatic ailments, while expectorants were logically recommended in respiratory diseases.

To detect variations in drug use among the practitioners in charge of the teaching ward, two of the most frequent disease categories — infectious and respiratory — were examined with regard to the prescription of purgatives and analgesics (Table 8.16). The data clearly show that all Edinburgh professors followed the same traditional guidelines and deviated little from the routine prescriptions. Fluctuations for the same practitoner in different years should be merely seen as responses to the individual characteristics displayed by their patients. Thus, no particular trends in drug prescribing surfaced from this analysis over the entire period of study, perhaps a reflection of institutional

Table 8.15: *Royal Infirmary of Edinburgh. Student casebooks 1771–1799. Employment of drugs in the various disease categories (percentage).*

	Purgatives	Anodynes	Emetics	Diaphoretics	Expectorants
Infectious diseases	61.3	40.7	47.6	35.6	23.6
Respiratory	57.5	53.9	43.1	22.3	48.2
Gastro-intestinal	80.2	49.4	31.8	17.5	13.1
Musculo-skeletal	61.7	49.3	28.3	60.4	8.6
Neurological	62.8	14.2	20.0	14.2	5.7
Circulatory	71.0	30.9	36.3	14.5	5.4
Skin	76.4	11.7	5.8	26.4	5.8
Gynaecological	70.0	43.3	23.3	3.3	13.3
Mental	64.0	32.0	28.0	8.0	8.0
Venereal	72.2	11.1	11.1	5.5	—
Urinary	53.0	52.9	11.7	17.6	5.8
Tumours	72.7	54.5	—	36.3	18.1
Average	66.9	34.4	23.9	21.7	12.9

Table 8.16: *Royal Infirmary of Edinburgh. Student casebooks 1771–1799. Differential employment of drugs by Edinburgh Professors.*

Professor (dates)	Infectious diseases		Respiratory diseases (percentage of cases)	
	Purgatives	Anodynes	Purgatives	Anodynes
John Gregory (71–72)	70.0	40.0	80.0	60.0
W. Cullen (72–73)	80.0	10.0	42.8	57.1
W. Cullen (73–74)	52.0	4.0	100.0	40.0
James Gregory (79–80)	67.7	38.7	47.6	42.8
F. Home (80–81)	50.0	37.5	60.0	20.0
J. Hope (81)	76.9	30.7	75.0	50.0
J. Gregory (81–82) I	52.3	52.3	42.8	71.4
J. Gregory (81–82) II	64.7	70.5	42.8	78.5
J. Gregory (85–86)	21.4	71.4	50.0	83.3
F. Home (86–87)	75.0	12.5	90.0	20.0
A. Duncan (95)	100.0	60.0	58.8	82.3
J. Gregory (95–96)	52.1	56.5	25.0	87.5
T. Hope (96–97)	40.0	30.0	36.3	36.3
D. Rutherford (99)	75.0	46.4	78.9	31.5
Average	62.6	40.0	59.2	54.3

pressures to streamline medical therapy and employ in-house remedies listed in the Infirmary's own dispensary.

Perhaps one exception was James Gregory, who consistently employed more analgesics such as opium and its derivatives in the treatment of both infectious and respiratory diseases. Gregory favoured the admission of patients suffering from 'typhus fever'

Table 8.17: Royal Infirmary of Edinburgh. Student casebooks 1771–1799. Physical methods prescribed in hospital practice.

Method	Cases (%)	
Blisters	285	(21.5)
Fomentations	188	(14.2)
Enemas	181	(13.8)
Venesections	171	(12.9)
Leeches	85	(6.3)
Rubbings	81	(6.1)
Warm bath	65	(4.9)
Electricity	62	(4.6)
Cupping	46	(3.4)
Foot baths	30	(2.6)

and 'pectoral complaint' during his winter months' rotation. These cases gave him the opportunity to demonstrate to his students the virtues of a conservative regimen based on rest, food and analgesics. Finally, Andrew Duncan, another Edinburgh professor, was known for his prescription of more exotic herbal preparations, but their alleged pharmaceutical actions coincided with those of the commonly employed drugs.[23]

Table 8.17 depicts the relative frequency of physical methods prescribed for patients contained in the student casebooks. While drug use failed to disclose significant changes between the sexes, some physical treatments were clearly applied with greater frequency to one gender than the other. Male patients, for example, endured more often the painful procedures of skin scarification, foot punctures, and the production of issues and setons. Men also often had their heads shaved if they complained of severe headaches. Females, in turn, were more prone to receive fomentations and foot baths, enemas, venesections, and electric shocks.

As with drugs, one can examine the employment of physical methods in the various disease categories (Table 8.18). As can be seen, blisters were most frequently applied in respiratory ailments, while fomentations were indicated in musculo-skeletal conditions. More than a third of all cases suffering from respiratory and rheumatic complaints were subjected to bloodletting. Leeching, in turn, was reserved for localised problems such as inguinal lumps (mostly venereal) and swollen joints. Finally, recommendations for the application of electrical sparks were issued in cases of paralysis as well as amenorrhoea.

Table 8.18: Royal Infirmary of Edinburgh. Student casebooks 1771-1799. Employment of physical measures in the various disease categories (percentages).

Disease	Blisters	Fomentations	Enemas	Venesections	Leeches	Electricity
Infectious diseases	32.6	31.7	33.9	22.7	15.4	3.8
Respiratory	64.0	12.9	17.9	34.5	3.5	1.4
Gastro-intestinal	16.4	19.7	26.3	9.8	4.3	3.2
Musculo-skeletal	38.2	33.3	17.2	34.5	22.2	11.1
Neurological	51.4	8.5	14.2	11.4	11.4	34.2
Circulatory	18.1	32.7	5.4	9.0	—	1.8
Skin	8.8	26.4	8.8	5.8	8.8	2.9
Gynaecological	23.3	23.3	30.0	23.3	—	23.3
Mental	32.0	16.0	24.0	16.0	8.0	16.0
Venereal	5.5	5.5	—	5.5	22.2	—
Urinary	—	11.7	23.5	22.2	5.8	11.7
Tumours	—	27.2	18.1	9.0	9.0	—

Table 8.19: Royal Infirmary of Edinburgh. Student casebooks 1771–1799. Differential employment of physical measures by Edinburgh Professors.

Professor (dates)	Infectious diseases		Respiratory diseases	
		(percentage of cases)		
	Blisters	Venesections	Blisters	Venesections
John Gregory (71–72)	55.0	55.0	20.0	60.0
W. Cullen (72–73)	30.0	20.0	57.1	85.7
W. Cullen (73–74)	56.0	72.0	100.0	80.0
James Gregory (79–80)	6.4	3.2	47.6	42.8
F. Home (80–81)	12.5	50.0	80.0	80.0
J. Hope (81)	23.0	46.1	75.0	50.0
J. Gregory (81–82) I	19.0	14.2	57.1	28.5
J. Gregory (81–82) II	17.6	5.8	57.1	50.0
J. Gregory (85–86)	21.4	—	50.0	16.5
F. Home (86–87)	37.5	37.5	80.0	30.0
A. Duncan (95)	40.0	—	58.8	—
J. Gregory (95–96)	34.7	8.6	75.0	37.5
T. Hope (96–97)	40.0	—	72.7	9.0
D. Rutherford (99)	53.5	7.1	78.9	15.7
Average	31.9	22.8	64.9	41.8

Unlike drug use, physical measures disclosed clear variations in approach among Edinburgh professors. This was especially true with regard to the employment of bloodletting in infectious diseases. Two practitioners, Duncan and Thomas C. Hope, shied away from prescribing venesections altogether while James Gregory remained a somewhat reluctant advocate of this method in highly selected patients (Table 8.19).

In respiratory diseases, the differences in approach were less obvious, although here again, Duncan still refrained from bleeding altogether. His preferences, however, could be seen as part of a general trend, since the casebooks disclose a gradual decrease in the frequency and amount of venesection ordered by all Edinburgh practitioners during the 1780s and 1790s, at least in the teaching ward.

Finally, clinical cases disclose valuable data about the effects of medical treatment prescribed by those managing the patients. In the frequent progress notes, therapeutic results were generally characterised as good, fair or non-existent. This 18th-century judgment was usually made by the attending physicians themselves based on contemporary criteria of clinical effectiveness. As such, it constitutes a valuable piece of information, telling us how Edinburgh physicians evaluated hospital treatment.

Table 8.20: Royal Infirmary of Edinburgh. Student casebooks 1771–1799. Results of medical treatment — patient profile.

Result	Age	Sex (%)		Occupation (%)			
		Male	Female	Labourer	Soldier	Seamen	Servant
Good	26.4	35	45	33	56	17	62
Fair	29.8	35	34	36	22	33	21
None	32.6	22	15	18	6	41	13

Not surprisingly, so-called 'good' results were usually obtained with younger patients, many of them females, and especially servants. By contrast, the poorest effects occurred among hospitalised seamen, frequently beset with chronic, rheumatic ailments that failed to show improvement (Table 8.20).

When tabulated by disease categories, these therapeutic outcomes reveal the surprising fact that infectious diseases actually fared the best, since in more than half of the cases hospital practitioners claimed good results with their treatments. Most measures were only symptomatic, and one should also consider the youth of such patients as well as the benign and self-limited character of their complaints as contributing to the success. The poorest results, by contrast, involved long-standing urinary complaints, especially those involving bladder stones and obstructions (Table 8.21).

Based on their own judgments of therapeutic success, one can rank the Edinburgh professors according to their frequency of 'good' results. Obviously such ratings are quite subjective, and they fail to consider the nature and seriousness of cases chosen for admission. Nevertheless, as a measurement perhaps of individual optimism and selective patient admission, the highest success rate corresponds to Thomas C. Hope who reported 'good' results with treatments in 49 per cent of his cases managed in the Infirmary's teaching ward, closely followed by William Cullen with 48 per cent. Professors with the lowest percentages were John Hope (33 per cent) and Francis Home (32 per cent).

Discharge from the hospital recorded in the student casebooks, and especially the label attached to individual dismissals merits a brief analysis. As previously suggested, lower 'cure' rates (56 per cent) — hospital at large (70 per cent), and higher 'dead' rates (8 per cent) — hospital at large (3.5 per cent) were computed for the teaching ward of the Edinburgh Infirmary. A possible explanation

Table 8.21: *Royal Infirmary of Edinburgh. Student casebooks 1771–1799.*
Results of medical treatment in relation to disease categories (percentages).

Disease	Good	Fair	None	Unknown
Infectious diseases	61.3	23.6	12.0	3.1
Respiratory	46.0	32.3	15.8	5.9
Gastro-intestinal	44.0	33.0	12.0	11.0
Musculo-skeletal	39.5	42.0	13.5	5.0
Neurological	5.7	35.7	42.8	15.7
Circulatory	20.0	34.5	40.0	5.5
Skin	38.2	53.0	3.0	5.8
Gynaecological	20.0	50.0	20.0	10.0
Mental	44.0	40.0	8.0	8.0
Venereal	5.5	83.3	5.5	5.7
Genito-urinary	—	47.0	47.0	6.0
Tumours	9.0	45.4	45.4	0.2

Table 8.22: *Royal Infirmary of Edinburgh. Student casebooks 1771–1799.*
Discharge status of patients hospitalised in the teaching ward (percentages).

Status	Total	Female	Male
Cured	56	59	52
Relieved	17	16	18
By desire	10	8	12
Dead	8	6	10

Table 8.23: *Royal Infirmary of Edinburgh. Student casebooks 1771–1799.*
Discharge status related to major diagnostic categories.

Diagnosis	Cured (%)	Relieved (%)	Dead (%)
Circulatory disorders	34	20	22
Gastro-intestinal	56	20	6.5
Gynaecological	43	26	—
Infectious	72	7	8.5
Mental	56	24	—
Musculo-skeletal	64	17	2.5
Neurological	23	26	13
Respiratory	52	21	9
Skin	62	17	—
Tumours	18	27	9
Urinary	17	29	—
Venereal	89	—	—

Table 8.24: *Royal Infirmary of Edinburgh. Student casebooks 1771–1799. Differential discharge rates by practitioners.*

Professor (dates)	Cured (%)	Relieved (%)	Dead (%)
John Gregory (1771–72)	68	6	8
William Cullen (73–74)	45	15	18
William Cullen (74–75)	71	13	0
James Gregory (79–80)	56	10	4.7
Francis Home (80–81)	65	11	9
John Hope (81)	54	15	18
James Gregory (81–82) I	65	18	5.5
James Gregory (81–82) II	50	26	6
James Gregory (85–86)	49	19	12.2
Francis Home (86–87)	67	11	5.7
Andrew Duncan (95)	49	26	6.1
James Gregory (95–96)	38	37	9.2
Thomas C. Hope (96–97)	68	6	8
Daniel Rutherford (99)	43	16	7.4
Average	56.2	16.3	8.4

for these figures was the selective admission of patients with more serious or complicated ailments who would make better teaching cases (Table 8.22).

Studying the reported discharge status in relation to the major diagnostic categories is also quite informative. Not surprisingly, the highest 'cured' rates correspond to the various 'fevers' admitted to the teaching ward. In turn, the bulk of institutional deaths occurred among individuals with significant bodily swellings, usually reflecting circulatory disorders of cardiovascular or respiratory origin (Table 8.23).

Although discharge labels were also subjective expressions of institutional achievement subject to administrative and professional manipulation because of their public relations value, one can again rank the various Edinburgh professors on the basis of their cure rates. From the available evidence, it would appear that William Cullen, John Gregory, and Thomas C. Hope had the best statistics (Table 8.24), while the fate of James Gregory's patients inexplicably changed from one year to the next.

Epilogue

Using materials obtained from an unusually rich repository of documents pertaining to the Royal Infirmary of Edinburgh, I have tried briefly to illustrate both the nature and range of analyses possible in the history of hospitals. As stated before, my goal is to stimulate the study of hospital activities inasmuch as they represent a central locus of medical practice — often truly the contemporary 'state of art'. These records offer much to the social historian searching for the role of such institutions in their communities, the economic and political roots of hospital authority, the fortunes of private philanthropy, the shifting ecology of disease, etc.

We need to understand better society's compelling need to hospitalise certain individuals. What were the reasons prompting such a course of action? Whom was the hospital really for? Why was the spectrum of diseases changing? What was 'proper' for hospitals to contend with? On the other hand, such evidence offers historians of clinical medicine important clues for understanding the construction and classification of diseases, relationships between medical theory and practice, and the clinical guidelines governing therapeutics. How do physicians establish disease entities? Why do they prefer certain nomenclatures? What are the criteria employed in the classification of diseases? More importantly in the field of medical therapeutics, how and why do practitioners continue to carry out traditional measures? When and why do they become more sceptical about their treatments?

In the final analysis, however, all these issues are of course interrelated and the documents here assembled should stimulate scholars to write a 'total' hospital history, a reconstruction of institutional activities that takes into account both external and internal factors that are always inextricably linked together. Quantifying part of the information and computing the data will allow for comparisons with similar establishments in Britain or other European countries and among different medical practitioners. It certainly is much easier to carry out this research in later historical periods for which more numerous institutional records have survived.

Hospitals, especially those of the 18th century, have been stereotyped as 'gateways to death' on the basis of anecdotal accounts and sketchy impressions. Let us place the debate regarding their activities and role in medicine on a new level of discourse and scholarship.

Notes

1. Among such numerous accounts are Hector C. Cameron, *Mr. Guy's Hospital, 1726–1948* (London, Longmans, Green, 1954); J. Bloomfield, *St. George's Hospital, 1733–1933* (London, Medici Society, 1933); Hilary St. George Saunders, *The Middlesex Hospital, 1745–1948* (London, M. Parish, 1949).

2. See T. McKeown and R.G. Brown, 'Medical evidence related to English population changes in eighteenth century,' *Population Studies, 9* (1955/1956), 125. McKeown's conclusions were repeated by several authors in the 1960s and then included in Michel Foucault's book *The Birth of the Clinic: An Archaeology of Medical Perception*, trans. by A.M. Sheridan Smith (New York, Vintage Books, 1975), 18. The 'death-trap' comment is contained in a book review by Lawrence Stone titled 'Madness', *New York Review of Books, 29* (Dec. 16, 1982), 28.

3. See Guenter B. Risse, *Hospital Life in Enlightenment Scotland: Care and Teaching at the Royal Infirmary of Edinburgh*, (Cambridge, University Press, 1986).

4. Risse, *Hospital Life*, 26–7; see also 'List of the original subscribers and other donors to the Infirmary or Hospital for Sick Poor, preceding November 1730', in Edinburgh Infirmary, *An Account of the Rise and Establishment of the Infirmary or Hospital for Sick Poor, Erected at Edinburgh*, (Edinburgh, ca. 1730), 19–30.

5. Treasurer's Accounts, 1769–1795, 1796–1804, Mss Collection, Medical Archives, University of Edinburgh. See also tables 1.1, 1.2, and 1.3 in Risse, *Hospital Life*, 36, 39, 40.

6. Royal Infirmary of Edinburgh, Minute Book, Mss Collection, Medical Archives, University of Edinburgh.

7. The information was printed yearly in the January issue of *Scots Magazine*, usually under the section 'Affairs in Scotland' or in the appendix. See table 1.4 in Risse, *Hospital Life*, 46–9.

8. Edinburgh Infirmary, General Register of Patients, Mss Collection, Medical Archives, University of Edinburgh. These 500–600 page folios are available from 1770 onward except for one volume covering the period 28 March 1797 to 27 July 1799. See figure 1.2 and table 1.5 in Risse, *Hospital Life,* 51–3.

9. See table 1.7 in Risse, *Hospital Life*, 54–5.

10. For further details, 'Patients and their diseases', Ibid, 119–21.

11. Ibid, 121–4.

12. See S. Cherry, 'The hospitals and population growth: the voluntary general hospitals, mortality and local populations in the English provinces in the eighteenth and nineteenth centuries', *Population Studies, 34* (1980) 59–75, 251–65.

13. Risse, *Hospital Life*, 125–8.

14. For details consult 'The patient comes into our hands: admission process', in Ibid, 82–9.

15. Hospital discharges are discussed in Ibid, 228–39.

16. These problems came to light several decades later. See Royal Infirmary of Edinburgh, *Report of a Committee on the State of the Hospital* (Edinburgh, 1818).

17. A complete list of the casebooks is contained in appendix A of Risse, *Hospital Life*, 296–301. Among the most important are John Gregory, Clinical cases of the Royal Infirmary of Edinburgh (Edinburgh 1771–1772), Mss Collection, Medical Archives, University of Edinburgh; William Cullen, Clinical cases and reports taken at the Royal Infirmary of Edinburgh from Dr Cullen by Richard W. Hall (Edinburgh 1773–1774), Mss Collection, National Library of Medicine, Bethesda, USA; Andrew Duncan, Sr., Clinical reports and commentaries, Feb.–Apr. 1795, presented by Alexander Blackhall Morrison (Edinburgh 1795), Mss Collection, Royal College of Physicians, Edinburgh.

18. See table 5.4 in Risse, *Hospital Life*, 264.

19. For details, see 'patient selection' in Ibid, 252–5.

20. 'Diseases in the teaching ward, 1771–1799', Ibid, 255–7.

21. Complete information on medical therapeutics at the Edinburgh Infirmary is contained in Chapter 4, 'Hospital care: state of the medical art', in Ibid, 177–239.

22. These categories were based on an 18th-century 'natural order', see Andrew Duncan, Sr., *Elements of Therapeutics*, 2nd edn, 2 vols (Edinburgh, Drummond, 1773), 8–9.

23. Duncan's employment of drugs during his clinical rotation at the Edinburgh Infirmary between 1 February and 30 April 1795 has been examined by J. Worth Estes, 'Drug usage at the infirmary: the example of Dr Andrew Duncan, Sr.', appendix D, in Risse, *Hospital Life*, 351–84.

IV

The Qualitative and the Quantitative

9

Madness, Suicide and the Computer

Michael MacDonald

The social history of madness and suicide cannot be counted among the central problems of the history of medicine. But both topics raise important issues that are highly relevant to understanding how the social institutions that dealt with medical matters worked and how laymen used medical knowledge, questions that have rightly attracted the attention of a new generation of medical historians in Europe and America. These subjects are, moreover, not merely colourful and revealing case studies. They also pose methodological problems that must be confronted by anyone who studies the history of disease and healing. Some of the problems are epistemological; others are technical. They are exceedingly complex, and many questions that might usefully be asked about historical approaches to madness and suicide are beyond my competence to answer. My aim here will be a modest one. I shall discuss some of the ways in which the computer, one tool of the social historian, can be employed by medical historians, drawing on my own attempts to use it in my work on the history of madness and suicide. I have deliberately avoided detailed considerations of specific software and hardware applications in favour of reflections on more fundamental matters. Most of the discussions of quantitative methodology and computer analysis that I have read are disappointing because they fail to appreciate the limitations and opportunities presented by historical documents. The character of particular kinds of records, like the texture of marble, must determine the tools that the historical artist selects and how he wields them, or else the results will be as ugly and unsound as an inept sculpture. This paper is therefore as much about the materials for the study of madness and suicide as it is about methods of historical analysis. It will consider in particular medical case notes and coroners' records, documents that can be used to illuminate the history of physical as well as mental maladies.

The history of psychiatry used to be told as a simple tale of medical progress. It was part of the mythic identity of the medical profession, one of the legends that might be employed to illustrate the superiority of modern medicine over the superstitions of the past. Although the praise-singers who retold the tale sometimes struck discordant notes, their recitations were very respectful. Michel Foucault's celebrated history of madness was utterly at odds with this tradition. Based on some slipshod research and a great deal of conjecture, it was a brilliant polemical myth that inverted the legends of the tribe.[1] Instead of a story of progressive enlightenment, the history of psychiatry was a tale of progressively greater oppression. Lunatics, who were supposedly regarded as irrational sages in the Middle Ages, were imprisoned in asylums in the Age of Reason and subjected to total control by medical specialists (who proclaimed themselves to be reformers) in the late-18th and 19th centuries.

Ever since the publication of *L'histoire de la folie*, in 1961, rival groups of historians have retold their versions of the history of madness and shouted imprecations at each other, like contesting lineages at an African wedding. The reactions of the spectators seem to indicate that those who claim a kinship with Foucault have generally told the best stories and cried the loudest and most telling insults. Listening to the cacophony, one might well wonder if the history of psychiatry has any meaning at all for scholars seeking a fuller and truer account of the history of medicine. It is occasionally difficult to recognise that the most important themes in both the old and new legends about madness in the past raise issues that are fundamental to the history of medicine in early modern and modern society — for example, to make an arbitrary selection, the relationship between elite and folk medicine, the beliefs that justified the varieties of healing, the causes of the rise of specialised institutions to treat the insane, and the uses to which medical institutions were put.[2]

Perhaps the most important question that the participants in the struggle over the history of madness have raised is did insanity change over time? Most historians of psychiatry have been philosophical realists: they generally believe that mental illnesses are actual diseases that can be identified in historical sources. They may grant that names of mental maladies changed over time, and so did the interpretations that succeeding eras placed on them, but they regard madness itself as a timeless and universal phenomenon.[3] The revisionists, on the other hand, are nominalists. They generally argue that mental illnesses are merely labels that authorities and laymen use to stigmatise certain kinds of unacceptable behaviour. It follows, therefore, that as the prevailing norms of society change, new kinds of madness are invented and others disappear. From this perspective, the history of madness is the record of what civilisation did to its discontents.[4]

Many historians feel passionately committed to one side of this argument or the other, but they can do very little to advance it. The fundamental philosophical issues on which it is ultimately based cannot be settled simply by producing more empirical evidence. Had Samuel Johnson kicked Bishop Berkeley himself, he could not have proved that the injured cleric was wrong. Clinical and scientific data may persuade us subjectively that mental illnesses really exist, but they do not defeat relativistic arguments based on phenomenology and symbolic interactionism. Relativism would be of little moment if positivism produced satisfactory accounts of madness in the past, but a kind of historical phenomenalism is, in fact, an inescapable aspect of any empirically sound explanation for the changing meaning of insanity in the past. Historians usually cannot study the insane first hand: they must rely on contemporaries' descriptions of people whom they believed to have been mentally disturbed. Even those of us who think that the psychiatric Johnsonians are right have to admit that the surviving documents interpose a translucent veil between us and the insane. The gauze of language, woven on a loom of convention by people whose concerns were different from ours, inevitably distorts our vision of past reality. To understand anything at all about the history of madness, we must examine first the patterns formed in the records themselves and the people and institutions that created them. It may be feasible then to identify maladies in the past that we recognise today, but my own experience suggests that the images of insanity in most sets of documents compiled before the 19th century are influenced so much by contemporary beliefs and conventions that retrospective diagnosis, while not necessarily invalid, yields disappointing results. A more fruitful approach to the history of insanity is to try to account for the shifting stereotypes of mental disorder by placing them in their historical and cultural context rather than to try to 'read through' them, as it were. This kind of contextualism avoids speculations from defective evidence and reveals a great deal about the attitudes of normal members of society as well as about those whom they believed to be insane.

In other words, historians of insanity do not in the first instance study the insane at all: they study observations of the insane. Any analysis of the data, quantitative or qualitative, must therefore pursue an approach to the history of mental disorders that emphasises the role of the observers as well as behaviour of the observed, and the viewpoint of the observers must be understood as fully as possible before any generalisations may be made about the impressions that they recorded. Historians must also admit the main point that medical anthropologists have advanced, that mental illnesses, like other kinds of diseases, are defined socially. Even if diseases have known biomedical causes, they are perceived and treated differently in different social circumstances.[5] Thus, whatever our views on the ontological status of mental illness are, it is essential to absorb some of the arguments and methods that have been advanced by the enemies of psychiatric positivism.

The simplest method of studying the problem of the meaning of madness over time is to examine the medical works for a given period and to describe the diseases and symptoms that their authors identify. This kind of history of psychiatric thought has been done often by historians tracing the origins of modern views of mental illness, and it has been practised more recently by historians seeking to relate ideas about madness to their wider social and intellectual context. It is the method of conservatives and revisionists alike, and it must be the starting point for any other approach. But the history of psychiatric thought tells us little about how the insane were actually identified. Until very recently medical experts seldom played a part in the initial decision to treat a person as a lunatic. Their taxonomies of madness classified the abnormalities of people who had already been labelled mad by their families, their neighbours, or by the authorities. An understanding of the meaning of madness in a given period must therefore be based on the ideas of lay people as well as the nosologies of the physicians. Ideally, one ought to study the psychiatry of both the 'great tradition' of the educated experts and the 'little tradition' of the common people and show how they were related to each other.[6]

Like most methodological prescriptions, this one is easier to issue than to fulfil. The common people's ideas about mental disorder were not expressed systematically. They must be reconstructed laboriously from fragmentary statements and from the actions of those who dealt with the insane. Some information can be gathered from popular literature, diaries, periodicals, and court records. But the most plentiful sources are the records of medical practices and of asylums. The case notes of some doctors who treated the insane survive, and so do the casebooks of many 19th-century asylums. These documents present one major difficulty: they were invariably kept by a medical authority. But in some instances it is possible to detect in them the beliefs and concerns of patients' families and sometimes of the patients themselves. In other cases, it is possible to compare the records of a medical authority with correspondence written by patients' families.[7] Even when the records are too sparse to yield a full picture of the attitudes of the patrons as well as the physician or asylum staff, they still can show how psychiatric theories were modified in practice by people trying to make sense of the behaviour of the insane. Medical practices and many early asylums were marketplaces in which concepts of insanity were bartered and compromises between the expert knowledge of the physician and the lay knowledge of the families and patients were struck. Treatment of the insane in such settings frequently depended on the establishment of a bond of understanding between the physician and his patrons, as Nancy Tomes has recently emphasised in her study of the Philadelphia Hospital for the Insane.[8] They were the points of contact between the great and little traditions.

The best records from medical practices and asylums reveal the pre-occupations of the insane and their families as well as those of the physician. Good practice notes contain observations about both physical and mental maladies, and there are hospital records that are analogous to asylum records. The techniques that social historians of insanity use to analyse such documents could be employed by historians of medicine to study the perception and treatment of other kinds of illness. The notebooks of the astrological physician and divine Richard Napier, which I used in my study of mental disorder in early 17th-century England, exemplify this kind of source.[9] They may be uniquely revealing in some respects. Napier's clients sought his treatment for almost every imaginable ailment of body and mind, and he recorded their complaints or the reports of their families sloppily but more-or-less systematically. He abbreviated what was said in consultations, but he did not alter his clients' words or impose a diagnostic label on their complaints. Sometimes he quoted his patrons verbatim, and he wrote a great deal of important and trivial information he learned during a consultation. The strategies and words of the participants in the medical marketplace are probably recorded more vividly and extensively in his notebooks than anywhere else.

Discovering the attitudes and opinions that Napier brought to the consulting room was a relatively straightforward task. It called for the familiar skills of biographical criticism. But analysing his clients' views and the common understanding of the meaning of mental illnesses that physician and patron arrived at in their consultations was much more difficult. Accepting the contradictions and imprecision of contemporary psychiatric lore, I studied mental illnesses first from the point of view of physicians and medical writers, the keepers of the great tradition, and then from the point of view of Napier's clients, the participants, if you will, in the little tradition. Using a selection of 16th- and early 17th-century medical texts, I made a very long list of symptoms that were regarded as the signs of mental illness or the psychiatric effects of physical diseases. I also collected as many descriptions of mad people as I could from court records, diaries, and literary texts, especially popular prose and drama. Reading Napier's notes with the language and images of contemporary psychiatry in mind, it was then possible to identify cases in which such signs appeared and in which they were believed by the physician or the client to have been psychological abnormalities.

I found some 2,483 recorded consultations in which at least one significant psychological symptom appeared. Several psychological complaints were usually recorded during a single session with a disturbed patient, so the total number of salient observations in Napier's notes is prodigious; perhaps 10,000 individual complaints are briefly recorded in them. Trying to identify meaningful patterns in thousands of short passages spread over almost 2,500 case notes is a massive undertaking. Some kinds of questions, such as the social characteristics of patients complaining of particular afflictions, could have been answered by simple counting. But interpreting the meaning of the symptoms themselves, ironically, required the use of a computer. A fast and flexible means of manipulating the data was necessary so that one could discover the ideas implicit in the thousands of symptoms Napier recorded. His notes were like pointillist paintings, composed of many colourful but tiny strokes, and the only way to see clearly the pictures of mental illnesses that they depicted was to look at them from a distance. Summarised in tabular form, the patterns of symptoms were clearer than they were when one examined each set of case notes in turn.

My hypothesis was that there were stereotypes of mental disorder that were used by physicians and laymen to recognise deviant behaviour. The notion that psychiatric abnormalities are not random but can be organised coherently into meaningful categories is, of course, as old as Western medicine itself, and it was widely shared by physicians and medical writers in Napier's day. The view that laymen as well as medical experts recognise stereotypes of mental disorder is perhaps less obvious, but it has been effectively defended by sociologists and usefully employed by anthropologists. Most of the questions that I wanted to ask could be reduced to a simple formula: what were the symptoms most likely to be associated with a specific symptom or social variable? I therefore coded almost everything in my transcripts of Napier's case notes, had the coded data punched onto cards, taught myself how to use the packaged programs available on Stanford University's monstrous IBM computer, and, finally, computed every tabulation that I could think of.[10]

The results were not entirely satisfying. The principal difficulty was that there is a conflict between the historian's duty to the evidence and the statistician's desire to achieve mathematically exact results. Like most 17th-century documents, the Napier case-books are imprecise, inconsistent and allusive. They were not kept with the needs of a statistician in mind. Even such basic information as the identities of the patients is often presented in ways that introduce uncertainty into the computations. It is easy to make a set of rules that provide a reasonable degree of assurance that John Smith of Milton is the same person as John Smythe of Moulton, but such identifications must always remain tentative. A much more serious problem arose, however, out of the limitations of the technique I employed to analyse symptoms, which was a variant of a well-known procedure called 'content analysis'. A content analysis of Napier's notes using the computer programs available to me in 1975 required the reduction of words and phrases to single numbers. But language cannot be stripped of its nuances and recombined numerically. Words shift their meaning in different contexts, and so even when I discovered a strong statistical link between two coded symptoms, it was necessary to review all of the cases in which the symptoms appeared to be sure that the coded phrases meant the same thing every time they appeared together. More often I found that although there was no strong numerical association between coded phrases, it was still possible to see a relationship between symptoms that were expressed in several different ways.

Still more vexing to the biomedical statisticians advising me at Stanford was the fact that few of the correlations between symptoms that we calculated were statistically significant. The reason for this was that there were a great number of symptoms (variables) and so each cross-tabulation (for example, of melancholy with sad) contained only a relatively small number of the observations being studied. Moreover, I steadfastly refused to merge consultations and cases into a few larger categories so that they would be easier for the statisticians to work with because all of the methods of aggregation that we discussed either violated the logical assumptions on which the questions I was asking were based or combined unlike concepts into single categories. Faithful to my training as an English historian, I insisted on splitting when the statisticians wanted me to do some lumping. Instead of mathematically sound bonds between symptoms, I therefore settled for a series of frequency distributions. Rather than analysing the data statistically, I simply summarised them numerically. I felt that this approach, although it lacked statistical rigour, was historiographically sound because it led me back again and again to the transcripts of the consultations themselves. The numbers in the frequency distributions helped to guide my attention away from the atypical and toward associations I would not otherwise have noticed. They were not really the basis for a quantitative analysis at all; they were a preliminary summary of a very fragmentary text that I then subjected to a more-or-less traditional style of historical interpretation, comparing the patterns of meaning I found in the notebooks with the stereotypes that were explicit in the medical books and implicit in popular literature and contemporary descriptions of mad people by medical laymen.

Much more sophisticated statistical procedures are available to historians who wish to use sources like Napier's case notes now than I was aware of a decade ago. Some kinds of computer modelling techniques seem particularly promising. But because of the complexity of language, I believe that content analyses like the one I carried out will probably always be rather imprecise statistically. Were I to embark on a quantitative analysis of such records today,

I would still concentrate as much on data management as on statistics.[11] Packaged programs for microcomputers now exist that would permit one to index all the significant phrases in the records and to examine them *in context* while one explored the associations between them. The data could be coded and statistical strategies selected *after* a much more systematic review of the links between symptoms than I was able to carry out. Some of the objections to lumping words and phrases together might therefore be overcome by the imaginative use of new technology, and it would be legitimate to employ sophisticated statistical techniques on the categories that one formed.[12]

Analysing the language and concepts in medical records quantitatively thus presents some very perplexing methodological problems, but a great deal can be accomplished simply by using the computer as a very powerful indexing tool. Statistical sophistication is not necessary to uncover meaningful patterns that would be very difficult to detect by shuffling and reshuffling note cards. For some purposes, assembling fragmentary observations into categories that can be analysed in the light of literary evidence may be sufficient. Most social and medical historians will not, however, use computers for content analysis. They will employ them mainly to perform relatively simple statistical studies of apparently straightforward documents, such as hospital admission records or coroners' inquests. Coroners' records are, in fact, one of the most important and least exploited kind of documents available to social historians of medicine. They survive in very large numbers from the 13th-century until the present. From the late 15th-century through the 19th-century, they adhered to a standard format and so they lend themselves to quantitative analysis. A typical inquisition from these centuries is brief and formulaic. It records the name of the deceased and the place and circumstances of his death, including details about the time of the fatal event and basic medical facts about the injury or illness. Some indication of the dead person's social status is usually included, and occasionally his age is also recorded. Every inquisition also includes a formal verdict as to the cause of death. Often the names of jurors are recorded as well as that of the coroner. Inquisitions from the 18th and early 19th-centuries that survive for some jurisdictions are accompanied by supporting documents. These include summonses to coroners and jurors, preliminary verdicts (sometimes with a note about the votes of the jury), and, most interestingly, brief summaries of the testimony of witnesses at inquests.[13]

A coroner's inquest was supposed to be held in the case of every sudden and potentially unnatural death in the land. A jury of local men was rapidly assembled when the coroner was summoned, and they were responsible for helping with his investigation as well as for bringing in a verdict as to the cause of death. Coroners' jurors were usually men of humble standing who were often familiar with the deceased or resident in the neighbourhood of his death. Expert medical testimony was seldom sought by coroners before the later 18th century. The witnesses who were summoned were laymen — the neighbours, kin and servants of the dead person and people who had actually seen him die. Coroners were mostly medical laymen as well. Very few of them had any medical training or experience: they were typically minor gentlemen or lawyers. An inquest was, therefore, an exercise in forensic medicine that was carried out by ordinary people under the direction of a man of some status and education.

A great deal of information pertinent to medical history could be extracted from coroners' inquisitions simply by tabulating the details in them. A much clearer picture of the hazards of everyday life can be got from them than we have been able to gain from other sources. The time and circumstances of death, for instance, highlight the occupational hazards that people encountered as the economy developed and diversified. The kinds of illnesses that led to verdicts of natural death or death by the visitation of God also deserve scrutiny. So do the basic social facts about the people who died from different kinds of mishaps: sex, social rank, and sometimes age profiles can be computed from inquests. Imaginatively interpreted, the results of such computations reveal information about a surprising range of topics.[14] Barbara Hanawalt, for example, has written a justly celebrated article about medieval parents' concern for the safety of their children from data recorded in coroners' rolls.[15] A similar study based on 18th-century records that include witnesses' depositions would be even more illuminating.

Coroners' records present some perils to the unwary historian. An inquest was a very complex social event. The judgments of the jury were influenced by their attitudes to the deceased and his family as well as by their medical knowledge. Some verdicts penalised the survivors by making them forfeit the instrument that had caused the death or, in the case of felonious suicide, the deceased's goods and chattels. The statistics computed from inquisitions must therefore be handled with extreme care. They are records of what the coroner and his jurors, who were frequently interested parties, reported to royal officials, not perfect reflections of events. The incidents depicted in them, in other words, are refracted by the beliefs and concerns of the people who recorded them. It is often impossible to estimate precisely the degree of distortion that affects particular kinds of data.[16] But even so, a careful study of the habits of juries can show how attitudes shifted over time. Inquisitions therefore provide an opportunity, and indeed an obligation, to study how lay medical knowledge was used in particular circumstances and how lay attitudes to illness and death changed. A good example of the possibilities is provided by inquisitions that record one apparently straightforward cause of death, suicide.

The statistical problems presented by the study of suicide from coroners' records are much simpler than those raised by the content analysis of medical case notes. Inquisitions are highly standardised and the quantifiable information in them is easily coded and counted. Huge numbers of them survive for the period 1485–1714 in the records of King's Bench; scattered sets of inquisitions and coroners' bills for the 18th century may be found in local records. My colleague Terence R. Murphy and I have been able to locate records of over 14,000 suicides reported between 1485 and 1800. Using an integrated spreadsheet program and a database management program, the basic facts about all of these cases have been entered on microcomputers and saved on diskettes. Very little coding is necessary using these programs, simple abbreviations are usually adequate, so the records are easily readable. As large batches of them were finished, the files are transferred from the discs to a mainframe computer at the University of Wisconsin–Madison, where they are abridged and revised so that basic statistics can be run on them using SPSS, a powerful and easily mastered package of programs available on many academic computers. On a smaller data set it would be possible to avoid using the mainframe altogether. Information could be entered in a form readable by SPSS and analysed by using the microcomputer version of the package.[17] Both the computer techniques and the statistical procedures that are required to analyse data such as suicide inquests are relatively simple. The greatest obstacle is practical: it takes a great deal of time to type several thousand cases into a microcomputer. For many purposes, it would have been adequate to have examined a selected sample of the data.

Ever since Durkheim, the study of suicide has been dominated by the analysis of statistics. It is a simple and revealing exercise to compute the suicide rates of different groups of people who killed themselves in early modern England. But the calculation of suicide rates is complicated by cultural changes that affected the meaning of suicide itself. Suicide was a heinous crime in 16th- and early 17th-century England. An offence against secular law, religious precepts and ancient popular beliefs, it was severely punished. A person convicted by a coroner's jury of deliberately taking his own life was declared a felon of himself, *felo de se*. Like other sorts of felons, he forfeited his goods and chattels to the crown. He was denied the rites of Christian burial by the church, and his body was desecrated, buried at a cross-roads with a stake driven through it. These savage penalties were stringently enforced in the century-and-a-half between the Reformation and the Restoration. There were only two ways to mitigate them. The jury might return a false verdict or conceal all or part of the property of the suicide from royal officials. This gambit was risky, though, because the King's Almoner could prosecute those who tried to cheat the crown of its right to the goods of felons, and the records of Star Chamber show that he guarded that prerogative jealously. Juries could, however, soften the severity of the law against suicide in another way; they could find that the deceased was insane when he killed himself. When a verdict of *non compos mentis* was returned, the suicide, like a lunatic who committed any other crime, was spared any penalty for his deed.[18]

Coroners' juries thus could choose between two different interpretations of suicide. One condemned self-murder as a crime like any other, a deed committed by a fully rational malefactor. The other excused it as the deed of a madman. Both of these interpretations were based on law and custom, but the *non compos mentis* verdict was also justified by medical theories. Many 16th- and 17th-century medical writers asserted that self-destruction was the outcome of mental illness. Robert Burton, for example, attributed it to melancholy, and he was joined by other writers in suggesting that mercy should be extended not merely to suicides who were utterly mad but also to those who had suffered long and severe melancholy.[19] Nobody before the Civil War was, however, prepared to advocate the wholesale use of *non compos mentis* verdicts. Religious beliefs exerted a much stronger influence on juries and commentators than did medical thought. Preachers and theologians stressed that suicide was literally diabolical, and they reinforced a deep popular abhorrence of the crime. The rites that were observed in burying the bodies of *felones de se* were meant to keep the spirits of suicides from troubling the living and to cleanse the community of the supernatural pollution that such a devilish deed left behind.[20] Throughout the 16th and early 17th centuries severity prevailed, and very few suicides were excused as *non compos mentis*. After about 1660, however, a remarkable shift in opinion and practice occurred. Elite attitudes to suicide became increasingly tolerant and juries began to return more and more *non compos mentis* verdicts. By 1700 they accounted for almost half of the verdicts returned, and by the reign of George III, they were virtually automatic. In the century-and-a-half after the English Revolution, then, the medical interpretation of suicide eclipsed the harsher legal and religious view. The crime was, in effect, secularised.

This shift in the meaning of suicide confounds the usual methods of studying the subject. Historians of suicide by-and-large still follow Durkheim's method of relating self-destruction to social factors. They try to construct rates of suicide for given periods and places and then to relate them to social and economic stresses. As sociologists have long argued, this method is flawed in theory and imprecise in practice. It is not hard to show that official statistics giving suicide rates are influenced by factors that make them unreliable evidence.[21] In the early modern period, verdicts of *felo de se* and *non compos mentis* were often brought in when the circumstances of the death precluded any direct proof that the deceased had taken his own life. The classification of deaths as suicides was, in brief, very subjective, and the procedure was often influenced by the attitudes of the coroner or the jury toward the deceased or his family. An overall suicide rate calculated from the verdicts of early modern coroners' juries would therefore be too inaccurate to be useful as a simple index of the health or sickness of the social organism. It would also be logically questionable. Different definitions of suicide with different practical consequences prevailed at the beginning and the end of the early modern period. Lumping all suicides together statistically ignores the fact that one is actually counting different things, the deeds of rational criminals and the acts of mentally ill people.

But if the changing definition of suicide must frustrate attempts to use Durkheimian approaches to the subject, it can facilitate the statistical study of cultural change. For the period 1660–1800, when attitudes toward suicide changed, my colleague and I were able to locate good collections of inquisitions that record the suicides of over 4,500 persons. The documents in King's Bench account for almost half of this total, and they cover the entire country. But the central government's supervision of coroners grew increasingly lax after 1660, and so the number of inquests returned to King's Bench declined. After 1714 very few coroners bothered to return their inquisitions on suicides to King's Bench. Almost 40 years later, the crown transferred the responsibility for paying coroners to the county benches, a belated recognition that the office had become essentially a local one. As a consequence of these administrative actions, records for the early 18th century are very sparse, but they are comparatively plentiful for the reign of George III. Fortunately, there are scattered troves of local records that cover the period, including a good set of 700 inquests on suicides in the city of Norwich, and excellent collections for Cumberland, Wiltshire, Westminster, and the City of London that cover the decades after 1760.[22]

Despite the discontinuities among the different collections of inquisitions for the period, computations of the verdicts in them display unmistakably the secularisation of suicide. They also reveal some unexpected clues about its causes and dynamics. Between 1660 and 1714, the proportion of *non compos mentis* verdicts returned to King's Bench rose from about seven per cent to 40 per cent and more. In Norwich the proportion of *non compos mentis* verdicts actually fell a bit in the mid-18th century, undoubtedly because of the influence of a particular coroner, but in the 1790s 94 per cent of Norwich suicides were declared to have been insane and there were no *felo de se* verdicts returned at all after 1770. Elsewhere very small numbers of suicides were still judged felons in the later 18th century, but well over 90 per cent of all verdicts from all the jurisdictions studied were *non compos mentis* after 1760. In other words, the evidence shows that juries treated suicide less and less as a diabolically motivated offence against God, nature and the king and more and more as an irrational act caused by mental disorder. The relative proportions of *non compos mentis* and *felo de se* verdicts were completely reversed in the century after the English Revolution. An examination of the depositions of witnesses in coroners' inquests in late-18th-century London confirms the fact that coroners and their juries thought that suicide itself was evidence of insanity by that time. The act was interpreted from the medical perspective and excused unless it was compounded by a greater offence, such as a violent crime, or was committed to escape the consequences of some other illegal or antisocial action.[23]

The secularisation of suicide was one aspect of a much broader alteration in the *mentalité* of early modern England. After the English Revolution, religious and magical beliefs that were based on the venerable assumption that supernatural powers and forces intervened frequently and pervasively in the lives of ordinary people were increasingly repudiated by the educated elite. Polite society condemned religious enthusiasm and mocked popular superstitions. Intellectuals embraced scientism and deism, and displayed, as Henry Halliwell complained as early as 1681, a 'hankering after the bare Mechanical causes of things'.[24] Many educated men and women and most of the common people did not, of course, share the *avant-garde*'s addiction to scientific explanations for events in this world, but the trend toward secularism in the century after the Restoration is unmistakable. Witchcraft prosecutions declined and then died out; most physicians and orthodox clergymen ceased attributing mysterious disorders to demonic possession; faith healing was abandoned to the Catholics, the sectarians, and the Methodists. The medicalisation of suicide verdicts provides an opportunity to learn more about the timing and causes of the demystification of the world.[25]

The shift in the treatment of suicides by juries might at first be viewed simply as an example of the adoption by men of middling rank of the secularist and scientific outlook of the governing elite.[26] Guided by coroners who were by-and-large minor gentlemen, juries embraced the values of their social superiors. But further statistical analysis reveals a more complex and dynamic picture. Examining the proportion of cases of felonious suicide in which goods for forfeiture were reported to the crown, one finds that the government's ability to enforce its prerogative right to the chattels of *felones de se* eroded even faster than the proportion of *non compos mentis* verdicts rose. Before the Civil War, goods were reported in inquisitions on about 40 per cent of all suicides. After 1660, the proportion of inquests in which goods were reported fell steadily until it reached less than 10 per cent between 1705 and 1714. Furthermore, the *value* of the goods forfeited also dropped. In the 1660s the value of the goods of self-murderers averaged about £6.14 but by the first decade of the 18th century their value averaged only £1.12. The ninety *felones de se* who died between 1710 and 1714 forfeited goods worth an average of just eight shillings. The actual erosion of the crown's ability to seize the goods of convicted suicides was even greater than the averages suggest. Throughout the early modern period most self-murderers were said to have had no goods, or property of very little value, but before 1690 royal officials had been able to snare estates that were worth hundreds of pounds in addition to the pitiful sums forfeited by most suicides. The largest forfeiture in the first decade of the 18th century was £99 and the largest in the next five years was just £24. Despairing Englishmen were certainly not poorer in the early 18th century than they had been during the Restoration and earlier; the crown's prerogative right to the pro-perty of self-murderers was simply being ignored by coroners and their juries.

Forfeiture had long been an unpopular aspect of the law against suicide. An examination of the surviving records of the Star Chamber reveals that the King's Almoner often prosecuted local officials and the families of suicides for attempting to evade forfeiture before the Civil War.[27] The abolition of the prerogative courts and the central government's failure to re-establish close control of local administration in the wake of the English Revolu-tion made it much safer and easier for coroners' juries to suspend the law. Commentators in the early 18th century stressed that it was sympathy for the survivors that led coroners' juries to return *non compos mentis* verdicts in increasing numbers.[28] The crown's declining capacity to enforce the traditional legal penalty for suicide can therefore be seen to have been a capitulation to a longstanding hostility to forfeiture on the part of local com-munities. From the point of view of the humble men who served on coroners' juries, the law against suicide seemed unfair, and in spite of very strong popular abhorrence of self-murder they chose increasingly to preserve the estates of their neighbours rather than to set the civil and religious penalties for suicide in motion. Paradoxically, the secularisation of the societal reaction to suicide thus began as a rejection by ordinary men of the civil penalties for suicide rather than as a repudiation of its traditional religious and magical meaning, and *in its first phases* it had little or nothing to do with medical and philosophical arguments. The timing of the change was determined largely by political and constitutional factors, for the events of the mid-17th century made it easier for juries to frustrate the royal prerogative after 1660. As the 18th century progressed, the secularisation of elite culture reinforced and eventually, in the reign of George III, subsumed the change that had begun on the local level. The belief that suicide was usually the consequence of insanity was gradually accepted by most people, at least as the basis for the community's response to such deaths. The demystification of this aspect of the mental world of early modern England involved not merely a transformation in elite culture but also the triumph of popular notions of just punishment.

The institutional locus of these very complex events was the coroner's jury. One feature that coroners' juries had in common with medical practices is that they were mediating institutions: they, too, were points of contact between the great and little traditions. Charged with summarising the evidence about a death into a single verdict, they had in their deliberations to reconcile different attitudes that were held by different groups. The pattern of forfeitures and verdicts in the records juries returned demonstrates that they did not slavishly follow the opinions of polite society. The balance of conflicting values shifted gradually in favour of the merciful treatment of suicides' families and eventually to suicides themselves. The forces of change are to be found in the undertow of popular culture as well as in the tides of elite opinion. The historian of suicide must therefore look beyond medical, legal, and philosophical texts, just as the historian of medicine must look beyond influential treatises and nosologies.[29] The statistical analysis of the actions of coroners' juries, like the tabulation of the symptoms of mental disorder, provides a tangible manifestation of the interplay of attitudes and beliefs. The numbers are like the shadows on an x-ray, forming imprecise and sometimes mystifying images, but interpreted with the help of supporting documents and literary texts, they can help us to arrive at a much more exact understanding of English culture and the events that changed it than we could otherwise achieve. Even cultural historians should learn to count.

The advocates of quantification often claim that statistical analysis produces results that turn conventional thinking about historical problems upside down. The assertion can be embarrassingly absurd: a statistical finding that is at odds with careful and expert reading of the whole range of evidence is probably anomalous and certainly possesses no special significance epistemologically.[30] But the claim is more often true than the critics of quantification will admit. I have tried in this paper to show that by using a computer to analyse medical case records and coroners' inquisitions we can greatly deepen our understanding of the history of madness and suicide. Used for content analysis or, more ordinarily, for the compilation of simple descriptive statistics, the computer reveals patterns that the historian would otherwise be unlikely to grasp. The assumption, prevalent in some circles, that quantification is incompatible with the humanist's traditional concern with language and context is wrong. The history of madness and suicide suggests that quantification can lead to a more subtle explanation of *mentalité* and of cultural change than simply reading the documents would. These case studies also highlight the need to practise old-fashioned historical criticism before reducing any of the information contained in documents to numbers. A thorough understanding of the people and institutions who kept the records we use must precede the application of statistical techniques, however simple. Arguments like the one made here that invoke phenomenology and espouse quantification ought not to inflame the spleen of historical traditionalists, for they are intended to justify a methodological tonic that is a cooling infusion of old and new ingredients.

The combination of both sensitivity to the meaning and context of records and mastery of quantitative skills is essential if medical historians are fully to exploit the surviving evidence about disease and healing in the past. The chief obstacles to using computers in historical research have been ignorance and penury. Most historians must teach themselves how to use computers and raise the money to pay for equipment or computing time. Like other converts to quantification a decade ago, I discovered that it was time-consuming and very expensive. Mastering very basic programming and learning to make the computer work were slow and frustrating tasks. Coding and entering the data I had copied from Napier's notebooks took months. When I ran the main programs at last, my research funds vanished with a speed that was much more impressive than the rate at which I managed to generate meaningful results. The rapid changes in computer technology of the past few years have greatly reduced the severity of these problems. Packaged programs for entering and manipulating data and for performing statistical analysis make using the new generation of microcomputers relatively simple. The time that it takes for a beginner to make effective use of computers has been reduced so much that it no longer ought to influence significantly our research strategies.

Quantitative projects are also comparatively cheap when they are carried out on microcomputers. Most researchers will find that the minimal requirements for a relatively large project are a powerful database management program and a computer with 512K of RAM and a hard disc.[31] In the United States, the price tag for such equipment amounts to several thousand dollars. But at the University of Wisconsin it costs almost as much to compile statistics on a very large data set using the mainframe. If they can purchase microcomputers, historians have more than a huge pile of printout when their statistics have been computed. They will also possess a machine on which they can keep their notes and bibliography, write their books, and do other projects. Cheaper and better machines and software have been developed at astonishing speed. Schemes that underwrite all or part of the cost of personal computers exist in some American universities, and it would greatly assist the development of the profession if they were more widespread. 'Knitting needles and filing cards', my wise British supervisor cried as I took my leave of him in 1974, and during the months I spent in the Stanford Computer Center, surrounded by preternaturally pallid men dressed in Bermuda shorts and sandals, his advice rang changes in my mind. I did not touch a computer between 1975 and 1984. Now, after more than a year of experience with a microcomputer, I can say at last that his words have a dying fall.

Notes

1. Michel Foucault, *Histoire de la folie à l'âge classique*, 2nd edn (Paris, Gallimard, 1972). For trenchant criticism of Foucault's methods see H.C. Erik Midelfort, 'Madness and Civilisation in Early Modern Europe', in Barbara Malament (ed.), *After the Reformation* (Philadelphia, University of Pennsylvania Press, 1980); Lawrence Stone, 'Madness', *The New York Review of Books, 29* (16 December 1982), 28–30; Lawrence Stone and Michel Foucault, 'An Exchange with Michel Foucault', *The New York Review of Books, 30* (31 March 1983), 42–4.

2. The literature on the topic is growing very fast. A sampling of important recent work on England should include Andrew T. Scull, *Museums of Madness: the Social Organization of Insanity in Nineteenth-Century England* (London, Allen Lane, 1979); Andrew T. Scull (ed.), *Madhouses, Mad-doctors, and Madmen* (Philadelphia, University of Pennsylvania Press, 1981); Roy Porter, 'The Rage of Party: A Glorious Revolution in English Psychiatry?', *Medical History, 27* (1983), 35–50; Michael MacDonald,

Mystical Bedlam: Madness, Anxiety and Healing in Seventeenth-Century England (Cambridge, University Press, 1981); W.F. Bynum, Roy Porter, and Michael Shepherd (eds.), *The Anatomy of Madness* (2 vols.; London, Tavistock, 1985); Anne Digby, *Madness, Morality, and Medicine: A Study of the York Retreat, 1796–1914* (Cambridge, University Press, 1985).

3. This position is especially apparent in the influential anthology by Richard Hunter and Ida Macalpine, *Three Hundred Years of Psychiatry, 1535–1860* (London, Oxford University Press, 1963). For an intelligent defense of it see Carol Zisowitz Stearns, 'A Second Opinion on MacDonald's *Mystical Bedlam'*, *Journal of Social History, 17* (1983), 149–51.

4. Foucault, *Histoire de la folie*; Scull, *Museums of Madness*; MacDonald, *Mystical Bedlam*, Ch. 4, which adopts a slightly different position.

5. Michael MacDonald, 'Anthropological Perspectives on the History of Science and Medicine', in Pietro Corsi and Paul Weindling (eds.) *Information Sources in the History of Science and Medicine* (London, Butterworth, 1983); Allen Young, 'The Anthropologies of Illness and Sickness', *Annual Review of Anthropology, 11* (1982), 257–85.

6. Robert Redfield, *Peasant Society and Culture* (Chicago, University of Chicago Press, 1969); Peter Burke, *Popular Culture in Early Modern Europe* (New York, Harper and Row, 1978), 23–9; MacDonald, 'Anthropological Perspectives'.

7. See, for instance, Nancy Tomes, *A Generous Confidence: Thomas Story Kirkbride and the Art of Asylum-Keeping, 1840–1883* (Cambridge, University Press, 1984), pp. 108–13, 191–3.

8. Tomes, *A Generous Confidence*.

9. MacDonald, *Mystical Bedlam*. Ronald C. Sawyer has completed a parallel examination of physical maladies based on Napier's notes and on documents from the locality of his practice: 'Health, Disease, and Healing in the Southeast Midlands, 1597–1634', unpublished Ph.D. thesis, University of Wisconsin-Madison, 1986. Credit for the 'discovery' of Napier's notebooks belongs to Keith Thomas, who discusses them in *Religion and the Decline of Magic* (Harmondsworth, Penguin, 1980), esp. pp. 362, 450–1.

10. Some historiographical analogues to this approach were available in the mid-1970s, and more have appeared since. See Michel Foucault, *Naissance de la clinique* (Paris, Presses Universitaires de France, 1963); Foucault, *Histoire de la folie*, pp. 269–315; Jean-Pierre Peter, 'Malades et maladies à la fin du XVIIIe siècle', *Annales: E.S.C., 22* (1967), 711–51; Jean-Pierre Peter, 'Les mots et les objects de la maladie', *Revue historique*, no. 499 (1971), 13–38. And for more recent work on English and Scottish sources, the research reported by Anne Digby and Guenter Risse in their contributions to this volume.

11. I am not here arguing in favour of statistical imprecision. It is frequently urged that the poorer the data the more complex the statistical techniques that should be used to analyse it. This may be true as a general rule, but linguistic associations are not the same as other kinds of correlations and cannot be meaningful unless the historian has first established that his units of analysis are coherent. For example, unless the historian is absolutely satisfied that all 'sadness' words really signify sadness when they are found together with the other symptoms with which he wishes to

link sadness, measures of correlation or association will be flawed, no matter how sophisticated they are mathematically.

12. At least one powerful text-management program is already available that would make it possible to perform simple content analyses on very large files of notes on a microcomputer: FYI 3000, produced by Software Marketing Associates of Austin, Texas. The program permits one to enter information with a word processing program and to index and cross-index it very freely and very quickly. It will also count keywords, which may be combinations of several words or phrases. The capacity of the program is potentially huge and seems to be limited only by the kind of disc storage device used.

13. Coroner's inquests and bills are discussed by R.F. Hunnisett, *The Medieval Coroner* (Cambridge, University Press, 1961); R.F. Hunnisett (ed.), *Calendar of Nottinghamshire Coroners' Inquests*, Thoroton Society Record Series, vol. 25 (Nottingham, 1969); R.F. Hunnisett, 'The Importance of Eighteenth-Century Coroners' Bills', in E.W. Ives and A.H. Manchester (eds.) *Law, Litigants, and the Legal Profession* (London, Royal Historical Society, 1983); R.F. Hunnisett (ed.), *Wiltshire Coroners' Bills, 1752–1796*, Wiltshire Record Society, vol. 36, (Devizes, 1980 [1981]); Thomas R. Forbes, *Chronicle from Aldgate* (New Haven, Yale University Press, 1971); Thomas R. Forbes, *Coroner's Quest*, Transactions of the American Philosophical Society, vol. 68 (1978), Part I; Thomas R. Forbes, 'Inquests into London and Middlesex Homicides, 1673–1782', *Yale Journal of Biology and Medicine, 50* (1977), 207–20.

14. Cf. Hunnisett's remarks on the more laconic coroners' bills, 'The Importance of Eighteenth-Century Coroners' Bills'.

15. Barbara A. Hanawalt, 'Childrearing among the Lower Classes of Late Medieval England', *Journal of Interdisciplinary History, 8* (1977), 1–22.

16. Michael MacDonald, 'The Inner Side of Wisdom: Suicide in Early Modern England', *Psychological Medicine, 7* (1977), 565–82.

17. A very powerful microcomputer would be necessary to carry out these rather simple steps on a data set larger than a few thousand cases: the SPSS programs alone occupy nine floppy discs. Some other statistical packages, Minitab, for example, would probably be more convenient and suitable for use on a wider range of microcomputers. For a smallish sample, say a thousand cases or fewer, an integrated spreadsheet program or a database management program and a statistical program could be used on a less powerful and costly system.

18. MacDonald, 'Inner Side of Wisdom'; MacDonald, *Mystical Bedlam*, 132–8.

19. MacDonald, 'Inner Side of Wisdom', 572–3.

20. MacDonald, 'Inner Side of Wisdom'; Richard L. Greaves, *Society and Religion in Elizabethan England* (Minneapolis, University of Minnesota, 1981), 531–7.

21. Important discussions of the reliability of suicide statistics based on coroners' verdicts include Jack D. Douglas, *The Social Meaning of Suicide* (Princeton, Princeton University Press, 1967); Steve Taylor, *Durkheim and the Study of Suicide* (London, Macmillan, 1982).

22. London, Public Record Office, KB 9–11, 29; Norwich, Norfolk and Norwich County Record Office, Norwich Coroners' Inquests,

1669–1800; Carlisle, Cumbria Record Office, D/Lec/CR I; London, Westminster Abbey Muniment Room and Library, Westminster Inquests, 1760–1800; London, Corporation of London Record Offie, Coroners' Inquests for London and Southwark, 1788–1800; London, Greater London Record Office, Westminster Coroners' Records, MJ/SPC.W, MJ/SPC.E are the leading collections.

23. Westminster Coroners' Inquests, 1760–1800; Coroners' Inquests for London and Southwark, 1788–1800; Middlesex Coroners' Records all contain depositions.

24. Henry Halliwell, *Melampronoea: Or a Discourse of the Polity of the Kingdom of Darkness* (London, 1681), 77–8.

25. Thomas, *Religion and Magic*, Chs. 18–22; Michael MacDonald, 'Religion, Social Change, and Psychological Healing in England', in W.J. Sheils (ed.) *The Church and Healing*, Studies in Church History, vol. 19 (Oxford, Blackwell, 1982); Porter, 'The Rage of Party'.

26. For opinion about suicide among the intellectual elite see S.E. Sprott, *The English Debate on Suicide* (La Salle, Ill., Open Court, 1961); Lester Crocker, 'The Discussion of Suicide in the Eighteenth Century', *Journal of the History of Ideas, 13* (1952), 47–59; and Charles Moore's magisterial *A Full Inquiry into the Subject of Suicide* (2 vols., London, 1790).

27. Public Record Office, STAC 2, 3, 4, 5, 6, 7, 8; MacDonald, 'Inner Side of Wisdom'.

28. See, for example, Arthur Wellesley Secord (ed.), *Defoe's Review* [no. 60 (30 September 1704)] (New York, Columbia University Press for the Facsimile Text Society, 1938), Book 2, 255; John Adams, *An Essay Concerning Self-Murther* (London, 1700), 29; William Fleetwood, *The Relative Duties of Parents and Children . . . in Sixteen Sermons: With Three More Upon the Case of Self-Murder* (London, 1705); *The Gentleman's Magazine*, vol. 19 (1749), 341; ibid., vol. 24 (1754), 507.

29. Keith Wrightson, 'Two Concepts of Order: Justices, Constables and Jurymen in Seventeenth-Century England', in John Brewer and John Styles (eds.), *An Ungovernable People: The English and their Law in the Seventeenth and Eighteenth Centuries* (London, Hutchinson, 1980); Peter King, 'Decision-Makers and Decision-Making in the English Criminal Law, 1750–1800', *Historical Journal, 27* (1984), 25–58; Cynthia B. Herrup, 'Law and Morality in Seventeenth-Century England', *Past and Present*, no. 106 (1985), 102–23.

30. The claims for the superiority of quantitative facts are advanced most uncompromisingly by J. Morgan Kousser, perhaps the leading American advocate of 'Quantitative Social Science History'. For an example of his swashbuckling brand of historiography see 'The Revivalism of Narrative: A Response to Recent Criticisms of Quantitative History', *Social Science History, 8* (1984), 133–49, esp. 140–1, 145.

31. The estimates of the requirements are based on my own experience with several hardware configurations. For some good, clear advice about software see Robert McCaa, 'Microcomputer Software Designs for Historians: Word Processing, Filing, and Data Entry Programs', *Historical Methods, 17* (1984), 68–74. Not all of McCaa's choices will suit everyone, and new products are available all the time, but the kinds of

programs he discusses are essential. *Historical Methods* is only one of several periodicals that provide software recommendations for humanists and social scientists on a regular basis.

10

Interfaces: Perceptions of Health and Illness in Early Modern England

Andrew Wear

One of the great merits of the contributors to this volume is that they have kept the individual and society in view. Despite dealing with numbers, populations, institutions, *la longue durée* and the structures of thought and behaviour that interest anthropologists, the contributors have seen their methods and conclusions as adding to the history of people and their health. Unlike the history of medical ideas or self-serving histories of institutions or of medical disciplines, the focus of the previous chapters has been on the ill person and population just as much as on the medical practitioner. Risse and Digby analyse the types of patient and their ills that came to the Edinburgh Infirmary and the York Retreat as well as the doctors and treatment. MacDonald's work on Napier and on suicides tries to capture the discourse and thought of the ordinary person. Of the 'French' contributors, Loux, with her anthropological training, chooses material for a history of health built up from the beliefs and behaviour of peasant society; Goubert shows how a total history of health and illness for a region can be written; Jones indicates the pressures exerted by students and clients — who today might be thought to have little influence — on medical training; and Gelfand discusses the *Annales* school of French history and its approach to the history of medicine — again one that has a wide focus and sees medicine from society's point of view. The two historical demographers, Wrigley and Imhof, show how from demographic findings one is led into general issues in the social history of medicine.

Therefore, although contributors to this book are eclectic in material and topic, there is another type of eclecticism that unites them: a view of the history of medicine that encompasses the whole of society, which uses a variety of methods to develop a new and mature social history of medicine and which is based less on theoretical dogma and much more on empirical research.

In this, the concluding essay, I will use some of the approaches put forward by the contributors and see how far they are useful for a study of perceptions of health and illness in early modern England. Not all approaches can be discussed (institutions, for instance, were few in this period in England); I will look in particular at *la longue durée* and the history of events in relation to the history of *mentalité,* and also at the usefulness of demographic history for my project. Additionally, the study itself parallels the other contributions in aiming for a wide social history of medicine. But as this is a concluding chapter, and I refer back to previous chapters, it will not be possible to provide the amount and range of empirical data that would demonstrate this.

Introduction

A history of the perceptions of health, illness and death in early modern England has to begin with people and with texts. It encompasses the individual's reaction to misfortune but also traces conventional patterns of thought and action that he or she could use. In this chapter I will move from people to the structures of thought that they employed, but I will argue that we have to preserve the individual's voice.

The evidence for the project comes from diaries, letters, autobiographies, travellers' accounts, doctors' case books, religious tracts, cookery and medicine books, etc. Although not 'history from below', it is history from the middle, the history of literate but often unimportant people. Their perceptions and reactions to illness may not, at first sight, be a very important topic: it is not part of the history of events in the sense of traditional political history, not does it engage directly with the major concerns of economic and social history. There is, therefore, the 'so what?' problem. More specifically, the project may look dubious to Anglo-American historians of medicine. It does not fit into standard slots such as the history of the progress of medicine, or less whiggishly, the history of medical ideas, of medical institutions such as hospitals or asylums, or of the relations of medicine with the State. But, in fact, the project is valuable because of its wide scope and focus, showing that health and illness in early modern England can be understood only by an eclectic use of methods and evidence. The period itself was eclectic in its views of illness, treatments, and practitioners, and the project is open-ended because it reflects an open-ended health-care system. It was a time when medical orthodoxy did not control medical practice, nor was illness depersonalised in institutions — people were ill at home, and hospitals were few in number and small in capacity. This makes it easier to look at illness from lay people's points of view, for their ideas were often as authoritative as practitioners' were. Also, the questions asked by medical sociologists, for instance, about patient-doctor interaction and power, are posed more easily in a period before the increase in the authority of the medical profession.

The project is concerned with long-lasting structures of thought and action, the *longue durée* of the *Annales*, and with the world of events such as changing religious views or medical doctrines (of the kind that Gelfand has discussed in this book); and, given an infusion of demographic analysis and contextualisation, it could come close to the 'total history' practised by Jean-Pierre Goubert. For the Anglo-American medical historian it gives new categories, information and perspectives. My forthcoming book may perhaps demonstrate this claim, but here I can only sketch in part of the argument.

Essentially the study of perceptions of health and illness in a society is a relatively new topic for medical historians. My approach is close to Carlo Ginzburg's type of history in preserving the voice of the individual in contrast to the anonymity sometimes produced by the emphasis of the *Annalistes* on structure and quantity.[1] The 'new' history, as characterized by Ginzburg, does include aspects found also in the *Annales* school: methodological eclecticism free from a central dogma together with an interest in long-lasting structures whether of geography, demography, economics, thought and action. But, more specifically, Ginzburg points out that historians have been attracted by the example of anthropologists away from old topics, towards areas of behaviour and belief formerly seen by historians as being at best 'marginal curiosities', together with an emphasis on 'lived experience' and the close reading of evidence.[2] A study of people's perceptions of illness in 17th-century England might be said to fit this type of history. It is not concerned with the great men and events of history nor with the progress of medicine but with a humbler type of person and with more prosaic activities. A close reading of texts such as diaries is one of its essential requirements.

People and structures

When considering the history of perceptions of health and illness there are great advantages in not generalising too quickly, in not immediately seeking the structures of thought or cognitive frameworks[3] that influence people. To begin with people is not just a sign of English historical empiricism or romanticism. Illness is a process, it takes place over time, inducing different thoughts, actions and interactions not only in the patient but also in family members, medical practitioners, ministers and others. Conventional, standard ideas or actions may be involved, for instance, a sufferer seeing illness as a punishment of God. Particular case-histories can help to delineate such ideas and to produce generalisations concerning them, but the process of illness has a holistic character (because of its changes and ramifications) that cannot be analysed simply as an example of this or that standard body of knowledge or actions available in the society. This can be illustrated by looking at some case-histories.

On 1 August 1660 Pepys wrote that his wife Elizabeth was 'not very well of her old pain in the lip of her *chose*, which she had when we were first married'.[4] With, typical honest selfishness Pepys noted on the 6th: 'home to dinner all alone, my wife being ill in pain a-bed — which I was troubled at and not a little impatient',[5] while on 31 October: 'My wife hath been so ill of late of her old pain that I have not known her this fortnight almost, which is a pain to me'.[6] Illness was not usually only an individual affair, it affected others, often in ways that distorted its original subjective meaning; Pepys' 'pain' was the same yet completely different from his wife's.

Here we are in a half-way house; we do not have the sufferer's account, nor the practitioner's, but that of some-one who could be closer and empathise more with the sufferer than could the practitioner and whose feelings and interests were also involved. There is both objectivity and subjectivity in Pepys' description. He observed his wife, her pain was distanced and placed as an item in the diary, yet the range and type of emotion evoked by Pepys was different from what a physician would normally express. Pepys' tone was personal and related to his everyday activity and thoughts — it was open-ended. A physician's account would usually lack personal detail and would be highly formalised to the point where feeling was absent.

In the reports of the London surgeon John Wiseman on his

cases of venereal disease his description of the patient excluded the patient's emotional responses and his own social interaction with the patient. Here is a typical case: 'One of about 40 years of age, having a *Herpes exedens* on his right brow, a *marisca in podice* and *verrucae* about the *glans* . . . I let him blood, and purged him with the cathartick electuary . . .'[7]

It is easy to see why medical historians have found it easier to deal with this sort of material. It is part of a circumscribed body of literate knowledge, not very diverse in any one period, and easy for academics to handle and digest into a coherent shape. And the objectification of the patient in physicians' accounts and in institutional reports and statistics helps to make the writing of history easier but also tends to make it more unidimensional.

The range of issues that can be raised by non-medical accounts of illness shows up when Pepys came to describe a recurrence of his wife's pain and the possibility of surgical intervention. On the 24 October 1663 he wrote:

> She hath also a pain in the place which she used to have swellings in; and that that troubles me is that we fear that it is my matter that I give her that causes it, it never coming but after my having been with her.[8]

Some reactions seem almost universal, transcending historical periods (the long *longue durée*?) and lay people, then as now, theorised about the causes of illness and, especially in sexual matters, would experience a sense of guilt (or was it here blame?).

On November 16th Mr Hollyard, the surgeon, was called in, 'and he and I about our great work to look upon my wife's malady in her secrets'.[9] Pepys, like many other laymen, felt able to take part in the business of medicine as is shown by his remarks conjuring up the image of an expedition of Royal Society *virtuosi* about to embark upon a quest of discovery. Pepys, probably following Hollyard, then rationalised about the causes of his wife's illness:

> and it seems her great conflux of humours heretofore, that did use to swell there, did in breaking leave a hallow; which hath since gone in further and further, till now it is near three inches deep; but as God will have it, doth not run into the bodyward, but keeps to the outside of the skin, and so he must be forced to cut it open all along.[10]

The humoural theory was easily understood and often used by the public. It could give a graphic and vivid account of events in the body, often in narrative form (note in Pepys' account the sense of change over time and the liveliness of the language: 'the great conflux of humours . . ., that did use to swell there, did in breaking . . .').

Pepys quickly moved from theory and the objectification of his wife's symptoms to personal feeling:

> and which [the cutting] my heart I doubt will not serve for me to see done, and yet she will not have anybody else to see it done; no, not her own maids; and therefore I must do it, poor wretch, for her. Tomorrow night he is to do it.[11]

In fact, Elizabeth Pepys' fear of the pain and her own and her husband's worry about people knowing about the operation and the condition, was enough to persuade (or to stop) Hollyard from cutting:

> she being in bed, he and I alone to look again upon her parts, and there he doth find that though it would not be much pain, yet she is so fearful, and the thing will be somewhat painful in the tending, which I shall not be able to look after but must require a nurse and people about her; so that upon second thoughts, he believes that a fomentacion will do as well; and though it will be troublesome, yet no pain, and what her maid will be able to do without knowing directly what it is for, but only that it may be for the piles — for though it be nothing but what is very honest, yet my wife is loath to give occasion of discourse concerning it.[12]

The message of this passage is obvious: practitioners did not dictate to clients, lay people were involved in medical decisions, and worry about social *mores* (was it a fear of being thought to have syphilis?) and the need for privacy could affect events powerfully.

This little episode may pose some difficulty for the traditional medical historian. It has perhaps too many strands: the client-practitioner interaction, lay and professional medical knowledge, husband-wife interaction, privacy, the body and outsiders, and the whole business of imagination, empathy, pity and fear. The text of a practitioner like John Wiseman is single tracked along a Hippocratic model that is easy for the historian to handle and, moreover, it has been part of the 'legitimate' material of the history of medicine — being the practitioner's story.

Wiseman's cases rarely have any significance in themselves except as examplars of his practice. But what is important in Pepys is the here and now, the emotion and the action of the story. Yet this poses a problem. The biographer and the chronicler of political narrative history feel justified in giving full play to the individual and the moment, but the social historian, who would be more interested in this type of material, tends to go for groups and generalisations. Ginzburg and Le Roy Ladurie have written on individual figures but in full-length studies. What is difficult from the point of view of the craft of history is to mix case-histories with general history when aspects of the case are not integrated into the historical argument and stand out in isolation. But if we want to grasp and retain behaviour, such as Pepys' pity, which does not appear to belong to any particular period, that is what will have to happen.

But, having made a plea for the individual case-history or episode that allows the variety of responses and actions to appear, it is clear that people responded to illness and death in learnt, stereotyped, ways just as they did to other events.

Many of these responses endured over long periods. The approach to death is a case in point. As contemporaries knew, and historical demographers have confirmed, the expected outcome of illness was often death. The old mortality regime lasted for centuries, and perhaps the attitudes to death remained as long as it did. Thomas Becon, the early English Protestant (and many others), eloquently stitched together Biblical passages expressing the impermanence of life.

> For what is our life? It is even a vapour that appeareth for
> a little time, and then vanisheth away, as Job saith, my days
> are swifter than a runner, yea they pass away as the ships
> that be good under sail and as the eagle that flieth to the
> prey.[13]

The rite of passage into the world of death was controlled and elaborated by that most pedagogic of institutions, the Church. In some ways the question of the sacraments that separated Protestants from Catholics was a mere epiphenomenon, and despite the very different political, economic and religious systems of, for instance, renaissance Roman Catholic Italy and 17th century Protestant England there were structural similarities in their approach to death. Both societies saw natural death as a public occasion and spectacle (just like executions with which ordinary death was often compared). The death throes of a Medici or a Stuart and those of their humbler subjects were objects of intense interest.[14] The requirements of a good death in both societies were that the dying person should be contrite, should welcome death and should be rational. This was how the death of a young merchant, Guaberto Morelli was described in 1374.

> Finally, realizing that he had been stricken by the plague and aware that he was dying, he provided for the salvation of his soul with the same care, requesting all of the Holy Sacraments, and receiving them with the greatest devotion. With good and holy Psalms, he devoutly recommended his soul to God. Then, with good and gentle words, he begged the pardon of all members of that household, recommending his soul to everyone, having no more regard for the great than for the small. Then, in the presence of the whole company, he accused himself . . . of having spent some 10 to 12 lire from the fund for his own affairs, and, as I said, denouncing himself in the presence of all, he returned the money to the cash box. Then he departed from this life, being in full possession of his faculties to the final moment. Together with the priest, he said the prayers with a loud voice so that everyone heard him. Then, sensing that he was at the point of death, he urged the priest to recite more rapidly. And by God's grace, having completed the prayers, he and the priest together spoke the last words, 'Thanks be to God, amen'. He closed his eyes and rendered his soul to God at that precise moment.[15]

The same stress on lucidity and a religious, contrite frame of mind can be found in Protestant accounts of death. John Evelyn recounted the death of his five-year-old son, Richard:

> . . . I persuaded him to keepe his hands in bed, he demanded whether he might pray to God with his unjoyn'd and a little after whilst in great agonie, whether he should not offend God, by using his holy name so oft, calling for Ease: What shall I say of his frequent pathetical ejaculations utter'd of himselfe, Sweete *Jesus* save me, deliver me, pardon

my sinns. Let thine *Angels* revive me, etc: so early knowledge, so much piety and perfection.[16]

Both deaths were public events, both were examples of a good death. It appears that here, in the act of dying, we have a common pattern or structure of belief and action that transcends the periodisation used in narrative history. Both Catholics and Protestants felt the need for the actor, the patient, to give a performance[17] of the holy death. The Protestant traveller Fynes Moryson noted in Wittenberg the inscription 'Here stood the bed in which Luther gently died' and he wrote when correcting this *memento mori* for tourists:

> Luther was born at Isleb in the year 1483 and certainly died there in the house of Count Mansfield where after supper . . . he fell into his usual sickness, namely the stopping of humors in the orifice of his belly, and died thereupon at five of the clock in the morning . . . the said Count and his Countess and many others being present and receiving great comfort from his last exhortations; yet from his sudden death the malicious Jesuits took occasion to slander him, as if he died drunken; that by aspersions on his life and death, they might slander the reformation of religion which he first began.[18]

Is this part of the history of medicine? At the time religious writers like William Perkins warned off physicians from the death-bed, yet ministers acted as providers of medical expertise. Religion and medicine were intimately linked in this period. Moreover, professional barriers that were lower then than now cannot be used to justify the medical historian not studying a crucial part of 'illness behaviour'.

The *mentalité* (or structure of thought and action) that governed the death-bed appears to have been pretty uniform, there were few if any alternative plays available for the actors in any one period, though, of course, as the work of Ariès and Vovelle demonstrates change did take place over time. The effect of this uniformity was to make the individual do the expected. There were social pressures (allied structures of thought) in the form of the meanings ascribed to the process of dying that ensured that the play of death was, if possible, acted out. The social stigma of the sudden unprepared death was great, and if the death involved the actor losing his or her lines then society could project its punishment, hell. In 1459 Allessandra Strozzi wrote how comforted she was that her dying son Matteo was given by God

> the opportunity to confess, to receive communion and extreme unction. He did this with devotion, so I understand; from these signs, we may hope that God has prepared a good place for him.

She added that not everyone was so lucky: 'for whoever dies suddenly or is murdered . . . loses both body and soul'.[19]

William Perkins, the famous Puritan theologian, echoed popular beliefs when he tried to contradict them at the beginning of the 17th century. He wrote that an incoherent death with 'ravings and blasphemings' and 'the writhing of the lips, the turning of the neck, the buckling of the joints and the whole body' was due to natural causes and 'comes not of witchcraft and possessions, as people commonly think'.[20] Perkins also tried to change the meaning given to the act of dying:

> we must learn to reform our judgements of such as lie at the point of death. The common opinion is, that if a man die quickly and go away like a lamb (which in some diseases, as consumptions and such like, any man may do) then he goes straight to heaven: but if the violence of the disease stir up impatience, and cause frantic behaviours, then men used to say there is a judgement of God serving either to discover an hypocrite or to plague a wicked man. But the truth is otherwise. For indeed a man may die like a lamb; and yet go to hell: and one dying in exceeding torments and strange behaviour of the body, may go to heaven.[21]

Structures of thought, of *mentalité*, can change, but the change is by no means immediate. It took a long time for illness and dying to lose their significations in the way Perkins wished, and to be seen in naturalistic terms. Nehemiah Wallington, in his list of 'Judgments of God upon those that mock and call Roundhead' of 1643 wrote of a knight of the North 'a great opposer of the parliament: in his ordinary discourse calling them Roundheads often drinking healths to the confusion of Roundheads'. Wallington noted with glee the conjunction between the knight's physical symptom and the names of those he insulted: 'Lyes now desperately sick (if not dead) of a great swelling in his head that he is now like a monster, his head as big as three heads: it may be his hap to die a Roundhead against his will'.[22]

Examples of this type are numerous for the early modern period. The idea of illness as God given punishment together with providentialism helped to give these meanings to dying. The focus can be widened to see whole towns and countries, when gripped by plague, ordering days of humiliation and prayer to take away God's punishment.

The ill person or community did not, however, only have available the single response of religion. Naturalistic causes of illness were widely believed in. People could draw upon both types of knowledge as they tried to make sense of what was happening to themselves.[23] When Pepys had earache he wrote:

> . . . both head and breast in great pain, and which troubles me most my right eare is almost deaf. It is a cold, which God Almighty in justice did give me while I sat lewdly sporting with Mrs Lane the other day with the broken window in my neck. I went to bed with a posset, being very melancholy in consideration of the loss of my hearing.
> Up, though with pain in my head, stomach and ear and that deaf . . . called at Mr Holliards, who did give me some pills and tells me I shall have my hearing again and be well . . . [24]

The two systems existed side by side, not just because of the social power and pervasiveness of religion but because the efficacy of both was uncertain. Religion was a matter of faith, but so, in a sense, was belief in the effects of medicine. Henry Edmundson in his jocular *Comes Facundus in Via, The Fellow Traveller* (1658) expressed this sense of uncertainty when he discussed the question of cure.

> It is a great Question what does the cure, the Vulgar will tell you the last thing they took did the cure, as the last thing they did caused the disease; Some Physicians will ascribe it to the rarity and dearnesse, others to the variety and composition, others to the fitnesse and order etc. others think it is not the Physick or Physicians, but Nature being disburthened returns to her functions by degrees, and men from weaknesse to a more cheerfull condition, from a long

hunger to a more greedy appetite etc. And some adde, that it is not Nature but the God of Nature which heals us, and as the Proverb is, God heals, and the Physician hath the thanks. It is Gods compassion on the poor man who contemneth no means but is without any. It is the reward of his patience. It is God's seeing his teares, or hearing his or the Churches prayers for him . . .[25]

There were no statistically based clinical trials to resolve such issues. A statistical, quantitative approach was absent from most of the medicine of the time, though there were exceptions (see below), and in the Restoration period statistical demography began.

This uncertainty gave a degree of freedom for the individual sufferer who could move from religious to naturalistic explanations or choose to use one or the other. In terms of *Annales* history both formed part of the *longue durée*. The association of illness with punishment and cure was centuries long and illness had been explained in humoural terms for more than two millenia. Political and economic systems came and went but from the fifth century BC to at least the 18th century AD the concept of too much of a humour collecting in the body guided diagnosis and treatment, for, to underline Gelfand's discussion of *la longue durée* and the world of events, medical knowledge was not reconstituted every time there were new modes of social and political organisation.

Religious explanations for illness were very flexible; the framework might be religious but one's interpretations — for instance Wallington's roundhead — could be creative and original. The humoural system also was very pliable. It allowed the ill person to construct stories/accounts that would explain why they were ill. Ralph Josselin, the minister at Earls Colne in Essex in the mid-17th century, wrote of eating too many oysters:

> There was a surfett with oysters, which though they did not nauseat my stomacke, mett with so much phlegme in my stomacke, and being bound they lay corrupting in my stomacke.[26]

He ate little but 'dranke wine, strong beere pretty freely and that carried them of, and my vomits had tincture of them (oysters) to Tuesday'.[27] Josselin's imagination could make up a story of what was taking place inside his body, and he used that story to make sense of his recovery (the vomits bring up the corrupting oysters and phlegm). The point is that he had freedom to construct a story in different ways within the constraints of humoural medicine.

At the same time as Josselin ate his oysters he developed a pain in his leg (it is possible he saw a connection between the two). He initially called it the 'sciatica' pain, he then developed red spots so his 'nurse and phisitian', Lady Honywood (fulfilling the lady's role of providing medical expertise) thought it was scurvy. Later he believed he had dropsy: 'my leg occassions thoughts of the dropsie', 'I have some hopes that my dropsical humour or what it is abateth. lord bee my health'. The death of a woman from dropsy 'strangely suddenly in a manner' made him anxious 'lord bee the god of my health; and preserve mee from all evill for I am thy dedicated one'. Another worry is that he could have gangrene: 'My sweld leg brake which at first occasiond thoughts as to soreness, gangrening by the blacknes of it, and following of the humour'.[28]

The lack of scientific tests and the inherent ambiguity of the humoural system, which allowed for many different interpretations, produced problems of diagnosis. Josselin rarely consulted physicians, in a sense he was a self-taught physician; as befitted a clergyman of that time he read a few medical books and his wife helped at births. Apart from friends like Lady Honywood, Josselin chose to rely upon himself when it came to diagnosis. The medical system of the time had its labels — sciatica, scurvy, dropsy, gangrene — but the question was which label? The existence of a large popular and self-help medical literature is a sign that lay-people often expected to work the humoural system themselves.

I think the historian should also look at what lay behind Josselin's, or any other sufferer's search for a diagnosis: fear and anxiety. Josselin, underneath it all, was anxious:

> My ill leg sweld very much with some pain, stiffness . . . it had great influence on my thoughts, god in mercy stood between mee and the thoughts of death and the feares of it, my leg issued a litle, I applied a searcloth . . .[29]

Quite simply the condition of his leg made Josselin afraid he might die, and his search for possible diagnosis was an aspect of that fear.

Such fear was not uncommon, we saw it in Pepys' fear of deafness (there was, of course, his well-known fear of blindness) and a physician noted in 1619 how two of his patients 'feareth the dropsy' and 'she fears most consumption or dropsy'.[30] What came first — the labels dropsy, consumption, gangrene, etc., with their overtones of dread, or the fear itself — is a moot point. Certainly, without the existence of a *mentalité*, a structure of thought, that produced disease entities, fear would have had nothing to relate to and take specific shape. But fear of disease, disability and death seems to be universal and to underline different theories and responses to illness. The problem for historians, as I argued before, may be that to look at fear of illness or other psychological factors is to say nothing that is specific to a historical period. But in ignoring such emotions, historians depersonalise illness, just as much as do the texts of doctors.

Josselin also had freedom to move between structures of thought as well as within them. He understood his bad leg not only be referring to naturalistic medical ideas but also to God:

A fine day after many sweet dews, the lord good to mee in his word, yett his hand against mee in john (his son) and in my leg. I own thy rod oh lord and kisse it, intreating thee to show me favour in all things, tis to thee I commit my soule.[31]

Although the ways in which people were expected to die seems to have had little flexibility — perhaps not only because of social pressure and beliefs but also because the death bed scene is relatively circumscribed in time and we have only the reports of the onlookers rather than the thoughts of the main actor — there was flexibility in the structures of thought that people created and used over generations to make sense of illness. Rather than hiding the individual, the emphasis by the historian on structures of belief, *mentalité*, collective representations, or what you will, allows the individual to emerge. Whereas traditional history of medicine with its emphasis on the history of events, on great men, institutions, humanitarian or scientific progress hides the sufferer in pursuit of its goals of importance, the history of mentalities can uncover both the idealised structure of thought and action as it relates to illness, and its practice by individuals.

Structures and Events

Nevertheless, the history of events cannot be ignored. To understand the precise balance at different times between religious and naturalistic views of illness in men like Pepys and Josselin, their reactions to the Civil War, millenarianism and Restoration religious attitudes and laws have to be taken into account. Moreover, structures of thought did change because of events, slowly religious views of illness became less strong as the Restoration reaction to enthusiasm set in, though, significantly, Dissenters still kept to the old ideas.

I have been writing with one eye on the other contributions of this volume and so have been circumscribing my material. I have shown how the distinctions to which both Gelfand and Loux refer (the world of events/*la longue durée* and the historian's and the anthropologist's view of history) help the medical historian to capture new material and insight, especially with regard to cognitive structures, and make it easier to do history from below or from the middle. However, Loux's and Goubert's further point is also pertinent. The historian and the anthropologist have to come together and merge the history of structures and events into one. This is perhaps more easily done for the early modern period than later when the history of events, as Gelfand points out, became so powerful and influential that it tended to destroy long-lasting mentalities.

The period and the topic are rich in events and personalities, and a history of health and illness has to include them as well as long-lasting attitudes and ideas. But, I suspect, this can only be done satisfactorily if one concentrates first on structures. The analysis of structures of thought about health and illness could take two directions. On the one hand, a search for further meanings of health and illness that goes beyond the simple dichotomy of religion/naturalism to consider ideas such as purity and dirt, order and disorder. These lie behind many conceptions of illness; for instance, explanations of plague involve ideas of dirt on the physical level (miasma from cesspits) and dirt on the spiritual level (sin). Again, ideas of what constituted a healthy environment were often expressed in terms of dirt and cleanliness. The propaganda that came back from the English settlements in the early 17th century evoked images of fresh clean air and water and fragrant smells, in fact paradise.[32] Order and disorder were involved in the harmonious balance of humours inside the body. The functions of these structures of thought may have to do with psychological control (for instance, of one's own body-images) or with power (the rich able to achieve cleanliness in cities or recreating the primeval purity of the paradisical garden and so governing the poor through the process of emulation). Maybe, but this approach like that of Mary Douglas, which relates types of thought to social structure, although interesting, is ultimately no more than guess-work.[33] The ideas on health and illness were so similar in different European societies (or perhaps the societies were so similar) that the conclusions cannot be tested.

Another tack would be more useful. We are used to rapid change in our ideas of illness because of scientific medicine, its discoveries and professional power and because of a pharmaceutical industry that creates a stream of new drugs. In the period before this, people made their own drugs from minerals, plants and animals. They might buy them from apothecaries, but just as with buying care from physicians they could choose to rely on self-help. Such a system necessarily recreated other aspects of people's lives. Popular books on making medicines were also cookery books. The humoural system itself was based on the universal sense of touch (the qualities that in combination made up the humours were hot, cold, dry and wet) whilst other causes of disease were related to smells, taste or sight as were the methods of telling good and bad food and water. A system of medicine that had few specialist instruments, that was open to laypersons both in knowledge and techniques reflected their conditions of life and modes of experience. This allowed for self-diagnosis and treatment, and for the patient to talk in equal terms with the doctor. On this reading, the structures of thought about illness — whether religious, naturalistic or concerned with order and disorder, etc. — were reflections and extensions of other sources of experience and life, and it is natural that they should belong to the *longue durée* since herbs, minerals, animals, the senses of, for instance, the need to judge pure water (given a lack of official institutions and scientific techniques for doing this) had remained the same from Greek times.

There was, of course, a great deal happening in the world of events, and the history of health and illness in the period would be incomplete without recognising this. The reactions of governments to plague, the histories of the Royal College of Physicians, of the Society of Apothecaries, the entry onto the stage of exotic figures like Valentine Greatrakes, the Irish healer, all add to the picture but also contribute to our sense of the bounds of the possible. Governments, like people, used both religious and physical means in the face of illness; through narrative history the weak professional position of different medical practitioners and the consequent strength of self-help and quackery becomes obvious, whilst Greatrakes was 'the stroaker' — employing what was possible, an every-day act in a special way. The history of events, although it helps us to see how structures changed — the Restoration and the lessening in religious explanations, the increase in medical commercialism and advertising in the later 17th century and the inclusion of medicine into the professional economy — in the end could take place only against the backcloth provided by long-held attitudes and ways of life.[34] Only with the coming of industrial society did the sway of *la longue durée* come to an end.

Demographic history

At first sight, it might appear that another theme in this volume, demographic history, is not appropriate for a subject like 'perceptions of illness'. A type of history concerned only with patterns of births, marriages and deaths would omit the thoughts and actions of the ill. Birth and death are events, illness is usually a process that lasts for some time. The former are more easily quantified than the latter. Moreover, demographic history, because it deals with large numbers of people, tends to anonymity whilst the type of history that I have in mind, which captures the 'illness experience' of people, is necessarily focused upon specific individuals.

However, demographic history gives the qualitative historian valuable insights into the context of illness in the 17th century. The discovery of short-term mortality crises, of the figures for life expectancy and of the movement in population numbers over the century have produced a picture of the whole population that qualitative historians working within the limited scope of diaries, books, political records and other literary remains could not hope to achieve. These results can be used to illuminate the general situation into which individuals were placed. Other results of demographic history that relate to health and illness include the nuclear structure of families in 17th century England (important for knowing how the ill would be looked after in a family setting), the higher mortality in London as compared with the countryside, the influx of country people into London to make good the city's losses (known since Graunt's time) and the localised nature of many mortality crises.

This said, there does seem to be a major divide between qualitative and demographic historians. For the latter are objective, while the former, despite protestations to the contrary, know that they are subjective. The recent and authoritative history of English population by Wrigley and Schofield, for example, excludes qualitative material. It has one indexed reference to religion ('religious factors, cause of migration, 471'), yet it is generally recognised that religion had important and close connections with illness and death.[35] Keith Thomas shows the converse approach in *Religion and the Decline of Magic*, where he uses hardly any quantitative methods, and his comments throw some light on why historians of thought and demographic and quantitative historians often seem to be far apart.

> . . . I have only too often had to fall back upon the historian's traditional method of presentation by example and counter-example. Although this technique has some advantages, the computer has made it the intellectual equivalent of the bow and arrow in a nuclear age. But one cannot use the computer unless one has suitable material with which to supply it, and at present there seems to be no genuinely scientific method of measuring changes in the thinking of past generations.[36] [though see now Mac-Donald's chapter.]

One way of integrating qualitative and quantitative history, and here I am specifically referring to the practice of demographic historians, is to see the latter as influencing the former. Experience, beliefs and actions, rather than being of interest in their own right, are explained by factors that are seen as the underlying constituents of history. In this version of the argument demography becomes the hidden hand of history that guides actions and thoughts. For instance, Michael Flinn, in his excellent synthesis of demographic history, writes: 'There is a very strong tendency among demographic historians to attribute the relatively advanced age at first marriage among the women of early modern western Europe to a recognition of the need to maintain the demographic equilibrium'.[37] Although this form of teleology can appear crude, it makes good sense in places; for example, the close connection between an increase in marriages and the aftermath of a mortality crisis (when bereaved spouses find new partners).[38] Moreover, the work of historians such as Peter Laslett and Arthur Imhof[39] has used demography to throw light on the life of past generations in such a way that we are aware that if we did not possess it our sense of the social history of a period would be diminished. Imhof, especially, has taken demography excitingly near qualitative history by arguing that the strength of religious attitudes to illness and death owed a great deal to the ever-present expectation of death under the old mortality regime. Wrigley also shows in this volume that demographic history can integrate numbers with behavioural systems (marriage) and conditions of life (the placement of towns, etc.).

However, for the early modern period it may be easier to join demographic and general social history of medicine than to use demographic results to throw light, as Imhof does for later periods, on changes in behaviour related to the incidence of specific illness. Historical demographers have found it difficult to give any analysis of morbidity in the 17th century. As Wrigley and Schofield point out, cause of death (let alone morbidity) was rarely recorded consistently outside London and it is very difficult to identify diseases (in modern terminology) from contemporary descriptions.[40] This was even a problem at the time for John Graunt who, when faced with disease labels that had gone out of use was not always sure what the illness was in his terms.[41] Lacking, thus, reliable figures on morbidity it is impossible to relate changing medical and health ideas and practices to the increase or decrease in the incidence of particular diseases (the exception is plague, in which the death-rate can be so dramatic that a rough estimate can be sufficient).

Demography and qualitative history

One of the characteristics of empirical qualitative historians, though it is always dangerous to legislate for others, has been a concern with the intentions and consciousness of the people that they are studying. If demographic facts were shaping patterns of behaviour, as Imhof has argued, one could ask: were people at the time aware of them? At one level this is a trite question, since no-one could ignore the reality of plague or famine. But many of the long-term trends of historical demography such as the changes in population levels and growth over centuries would not have been perceived by 'men' who 'lived lives in a moving present and short-term prospects occupied most of their attention'.[42] However, the 17th century was the period when Graunt and Petty founded demography. Records in the form of parish registrations and the bills of mortality had been kept since the 16th century. English society had an incipient sense of demography even before Graunt (despite most historians' view that the birth of statistics, probability and demography was a sudden event of the 1660s[43]). This could take an unformed shape, for instance, in the frequent advice to avoid marshy ground, which now is being seen by demographers as well-founded in terms of the mortality of these places.[44] Aubrey noted that:

> Gilbert Sheldon, Lord Bishop of London, gave Dr Pell the scurvy Parsonage of Lanedon cum Basseldon in the infamous and unhealthy (aguesh) Hundreds of Essex (they call it killpriest sarcastically) and King Charles the Second gave him the Parsonage of Fobing, 4 miles distant.
>
> At Fobing, seven curates died within the first ten years; in sixteen years, six of those that had been his curates at Laidon are dead; besides those that went away from both places; and the death of his wife, servants and grand-children.[45]

A clear-cut demographic argument was used by the propagandists for the American settlements when they tried to entice money and settlers. They pointed out that the healthiness of a settlement could be judged by the survival rate amongst the settlers (of course the statistics were always favourable, any illnesses being declared to have been contracted before the voyage).[46] This type of argument was employed in the beginning of the 17th century and contradicts Hacking's view that before 1660 quantity was never used as an independent criterion to decide an issue.

Moreover, although short-term mortality crises are one of the major discoveries of modern historical demography, they were implicitly recognised by 17th century people and incorporated into their religious/knowledge system. The 'three arrows of God' were pestilence, war and famine, which today are considered the causes of short-term mortality crises. Church and State recognised them by setting aside special days of prayer and humiliation for such events.

Individuals like Ralph Josselin experienced and were aware of the local nature of plague epidemics. Josselin experienced dislocation consequent to war and was aware of the dearth following military movements. He also wrote explicitly of the economic consequences of bad harvests, especially the increase in prices and in debt. In all this he was to be echoed by historical demographers.

There clearly was some demographic knowledge in the society, and those within it were able to use quantitative arguments, so the power of demographic realities to shape people's behaviour should be acceptable to qualitative historians. Though both they and historical demographers have to be aware that quantification and demography had less significance in contemporary minds than they do now. When John Winthrop, the governor of Massachusetts, noted the wholesale destruction of the Indians by smallpox, he rejoiced in God's providence that confirmed the settlers' title to the land.[47] He showed no interest in relating the demographic facts to the illness and in wondering why smallpox was more fatal to the Indians than to his men.

The advice literature on health and illness lacked a demographic or quantitative element. Its style was aphoristic and assertive, and numbers were not used to decide between possible alternatives or on the success rate of the advice given. For instance, Everard Maynwaring in his *Tutela Sanitatis* . . . *The Protection of Long Life* advised 'Refuse Lambe, Kid, fresh Pork, Pig, Goose, Duck and water Fowle, being over moist and clogging a phlegmatick stomach'.[48] The only justification for this bald assertion is the reference to the very pliable humoural system, which, by metaphor and analogy, could graphically connect diverse subjects together (the moist lamb clogging a phlegmatic stomach). The only quasi-numerical justification found in the advice books derived from personal experience. Robert Wittie's *Scarbrough Spaw* (1660) was based on twenty-two years of observation of the effects of the medicinal spring 'not only in my selfe, but in very many others'.[49] Wittie gave no numbers and even if he had it would have been in terms of his experience (personal experience was one of the new criteria of knowledge), which was of necessity adventitious and limited. In a sense, humoural reasoning with its graphic, story-telling quality was the way by which advice on health gained conviction, and humoural narrative, with its emphasis on qualitative changes of bodily substances, was inimical to quantification. Wittie wrote 'Nor do I approve of drinking all of the Spaw in the afternoon . . . (because also it may) fly into the habit of the body and breed the Gout or some other moist disease of the joints'.[50] This type of reasoning, although apparently sure of itself, because of its subjective nature, was always liable to doubt. The sense of number did not exist when it came to individuals' accounts and explanations of their illness (today this might be one's blood pressure level or the chances of dying of lung cancer if a smoker) or to justification for particular pieces of medical advice. But a sense of number did exist as it related to certain types of illness and disaster where it found its greatest expression in plague, the bills of mortality and government responses. Paul Slack's *The Impact of Plague in Tudor and Stuart England* is but the latest example of how easy it is for the historian of plague to integrate demographic findings with the social and political history of the time, for governments and people acted on the demographic information available to them.

The work of John Graunt is a good end point, for it shows how little and how much historical demography has changed over the years. Like modern writers, Graunt played down, for practical reasons, diagnosis of causes of death in this period. The inexperience of the untrained searchers and the too great refinements of physicians' terminology led Graunt to take a broad view in which a label like sudden death was more important than 'apoplexy', 'planet struck', 'suddenly', etc. and where 'it is enough, if we know from the Searchers but the most predominant symptoms'.[51]

Graunt, however, not only forms a link with present day demography, he was also interested in peoples' views on illness. He included qualitative material such as fear, writing that 'many persons live in great fear and apprehension of the more formidable and notorious Diseases following . . .'[52] He then listed the numbers dying from such diseases so that the chances for any one person of dying in the future from one of them could be calculated. Despite some difficulties with changing disease labels, Graunt perhaps was able to include such material because the problems of understanding 17th century disease terminology were not so difficult as they are today — he had to take into account only changes that had occurred in the previous fifty years or so. Nevertheless, the subjective-objective, qualitative-quantitative divide was not as strong in Graunt as it became in later years. What is heartening is that historical demographers, whilst keeping to the objective core of their discipline, are now again, as this volume shows, prepared to enter the ambiguous territory between subjective thought and objective fact. In so doing they integrate their discipline into general history and, more particularly for this essay, they can follow the example of Imhof and contribute to the social history of health and illness and its mentalities. Just as there are interfaces within cognitive structures and between structures and events, so there are interfaces· between the numbers of demography and the thought and actions of people that will reward exploration.

Notes

1. Carlo Ginzburg, *The Cheese and the Worms* (London, Routledge and Kegan Paul, 1981), xx–xxii.

2. Carlo Ginzburg, 'Anthropology and History in the 1980s. A Comment' in T. Rabb and R.I. Rotberg, *The new History, the 1980s and Beyond* (Princeton, Princeton University Press, 1982), 227.

3. I have deliberately used the terms *mentalité*, 'cognitive frameworks', 'structures of thought' in a loose and interchangeable way, and I have blurred the distinction between the form and contents of thought. If readers feel that there is a danger of reifying thought by using such terms, I hope they will realise that much of this paper shows that structures of thought only have a reality when put into practice.

4. Samuel Pepys, *The Diary of Samuel Pepys*, Robert Latham, William Matthews (eds) (11 vols, London, Bell and Hyman, 1970–83), vol. 1, 213.

5. Ibid., p. 216.

6. Ibid., p. 279.

7. Richard Wiseman, *Severall Chirurgicall Treatises* (London, 1676), Book 7, 33.

8. Pepys, *Diary*, vol. 4, p. 347.

9. Ibid., p. 383.

10. Ibid., p. 383–4.

11. Ibid., p. 384.

12. Ibid., p. 385.

13. Thomas Becon, *The Sicke Mans Salve* (London 1561), p. 305.

14. See the description of the death-bed scene of Lorenzo de Medici in Janet Ross, *Lives of the early Medici as told in their Correspondence* (London, Chatto and Windus, 1910), 336–9; the reports of the death of Elizabeth in John Manningham, *The Diary of John Manningham*, R.P. Sorlien (ed.) (Hanover, R.I., University of Rhode Island, 1976), 207–8; reports of the death of Charles II in Edward Maunde Thompson, *Correspondence of the Family of Hatton*, (2 vols. Camden Society, New Series xxii–xxiii, 1878), vol. 2 51–4.

15. Gene Brucker (ed.) *The Society of Renaissance Florence. A Documentary Study* (New York, Harper Torchbooks, 1971), 46–7.

16. John Evelyn, *The Diary of John Evelyn*, E.S. de Beer (ed.) (6 vols, Oxford, University Press, 1955), vol. 3, 208.

17. Elizabeth, Countess of Bridgewater, wrote in her 'devotional pieces' collected in 1663 of the death of her daughter Kate: 'her life and death was nothing but sweetness, shewing us what we should perform on our last day'. British Library, Egerton MS 607, fol. 126v.

18. Fynes Moryson, *An Itinerary*, (4 vols, Glasgow, James MacLehose, 1907), vol. 1, 15.

19. Brucker, *The Society of Renaissance Florence*, p. 48.

20. William Perkins, 'The Right Way of Dying Well', in *A Golden Chaine* (London, 1612), 492.

21. Ibid., p. 492.

22. Nehemiah Wallington, British Library, Sloane MS 1457, fol. 71v.

23. See A. Wear, 'Puritan Perceptions of Illness in Seventeenth Century England' in R. Porter (ed.) *Patients and Practitioners* (Cambridge, University Press, 1985), 55–99.

24. Pepys, *Diary*, vol. 4, 318–19.

25. Henry Edmundson, *Comes Facundus in Via — The Fellow Traveller*, (London, 1658), 111–12.

26. R. Josselin, *The Diary of Ralph Josselin 1616–1683*, Alan Macfarlane (ed.) (London, British Academy, 1976), 566. Lucinda Beier has a chapter on Josselin in R. Porter's *Patients and Practitioners* and I have a page or two. See also Alan Macfarlane, *The Family Life of Ralph Josselin, An Essay in Historical Anthropology* (Cambridge, University Press, 1970).

27. Josselin, *Diary*, p. 566.

28. Ibid., p. 566, 572, 578, 582–3, 584.

29. Ibid., p. 584.

30. Anon., 'Diarium Practicum 1619–1622', British Library, Sloane 1112:1, p.1v.

31. Josselin, *Diary*, p. 585.

32. See H.C. Porter, *The Inconstant Savage, England and the North American Indian 1500–1660* (London, Duckworth, 1979); John Prest, *The Garden of Eden: The Botanical Garden and the Re-Creation of Paradise* (New Haven, Yale University Press, 1981); A. Wear, 'Perceptions of Health and the Environment in the Settlement of North American in the Early Seventeenth Century', *Bulletin of the Society for the Social History of Medicine*, *35*, (1984), 11–13.

33. Mary Douglas, *Purity and Danger* (Routledge and Kegan Paul, London, 1966) and *Natural Symbols: Explorations in Cosmology*, (Barrie and Rockcliff, London, 1970). There is a useful discussion of Douglas' ideas as they relate to the history of science by David Oldroyd, 'Grid Group Analysis for Historians of Science?', *History of Science, 24* (1986), 145–71. It is peculiar that historians of medicine have not taken up Douglas' ideas, material from the history of medicine is much closer to Douglas' evidence (pollution, hygiene) and the opportunity for seeing whether refutation of her views is possible is far greater.

34. Just as structures of thought only exist when they are put into practice by people, so they change when people, groups, governments, etc. choose to change them. The question of how the *longue durée* changes has been made to appear difficult by a tendency to idealise it.

35. E.A. Wrigley and R.S. Schofield, *The Population History of England 1541–1871: A Reconstruction* (London, Arnold, 1981); though the work does assume that people's hopes and fears as reflected in the rise and fall of prices, etc. do affect the birth rate.

36. Keith Thomas, *Religion and the Decline of Magic* (Harmondsworth, Penguin Books, 1973), p. x.

37. Michael W. Flinn, *The European Demographic System 1500–1820,* (Brighton, Harvester Press, 1981), p. 28.

38. Ibid., p. 34.

39. Peter Laslett, *The World We Have Lost — Further Explored* (London, Methuen, 1983); Arthur Imhof, *Die Verlorenen Welten* (Munich, Beck, 1984).

40. Wrigley and Schofield, *The Population History of England*, pp. 667–9.

41. John Graunt, *Natural and Political Observations . . . upon the Bills of Mortality*, 5th edn (London, 1676), 40: 'The Tyssick seems to be quite worn away, but that is probable the same is entered as "Cough" or "Consumption"'. However, *new* diseases also could be difficult to understand see, for instance, pp. 37–8 the 'new disease called by our Bills "The Stopping of the Stomach"'. Graunt wondered if this was the 'Green-sickness', or the 'Mother' or 'the Rising of the Lights'.

42. E.A. Wrigley, *Population and History* (London, Weidenfeld and Nicolson, 1969), 77–8.

43. On the early history of demography and statistics see Karl Pearson, E.S. Pearson (ed.) *The History of Statistics in the 17th and 18th Centuries* (London, 1978); I. Hacking, *The Emergence of Probability*, (Cambridge, University Press, 1975); James H. Cassedy, 'Medicine and the Rise of Statistics', in A.G. Debus (ed.) *Medicine in Seventeenth Century England* (Berkeley, University of California Press, 1974), 283–312; Ulrich Tröhler 'Quantification in British Medicine and Surgery 1750–1830', unpublished Ph.D. thesis, University of London, 1978, pp. 44–8. For a general discussion of the growth of a sense of number see Alexander Murray, *Reason and Society in the Middle Ages* (Oxford, University Press, 1978).

44. See Mary Dobson, 'Population, Disease, and Mortality in Southeast England 1600–1800'; unpublished D.Phil, Oxford University, 1982.

45. John Aubrey, *Aubrey's Brief Lives*, Oliver Lawson Dick (ed.) (London, 1975), 231.

46. See, for instance, Peter Force (ed.), *A plain Description of the Barmudas now called Sommer Ilands*, reprinted in *Tracts and Other Papers relating Principally to the Origin, Settlement and Progress of the Colonies in North America*, 4 vols, (Washington, 1836, reprint New York, Peter Smith, 1947), 111, 21 which describes three men left behind on the Island: the climate was good 'and agreeable with our constitutions of England, and for the victual very wholesome and good: for the three men which were left there are very fat and faire, not tanned or burned in the Sun so much as we which came last, and they say themselves they never were sicke all the time of their being there and one of them have been there three yeares and upwards'. More 'significant' perhaps was Thomas Hariot's *A Brief and True Report of Virginia* (London, 1588), which describes Raleigh's Roanake expedition. Hariot pointed out, p. 3v, that the expedition had been mainly

living 'by drinking water and by the victual of the country, of which some sorts were very strange unto us and might have been thought to have altered our temperatures [i.e. temperatures, bodily constitutions] in some sort as to have brought us into some grievous and dangerous diseases'. However, despite this and having to live in winter in the open air and to sleep on the ground, only four of the 108 died and three of them were 'feeble weake and sickly persons before ever they came thither'.

47. 'For the natives, they are near all dead of the smallpox, so as the Lord hath cleared our title to what we possess', John Winthrop to Sir Nathaniel Rich, May 22, 1634, in Everett Emerson (ed.) *Letters from New England* (Amherst, University of Massachusetts Press, 1976), p. 116.

48. Everard Maynwaring, *Tutela Sanitatis . . . The Protection of Long Life* (London, 1663), p. 42.

49. Robert Wittie, *Scarborough Spaw or a Description of the Nature and Virtues of the Spaw at Scarborough in Yorkshire . . .* (London, 1660), p. 8.

50. Ibid., p. 228.

51. Graunt, *Natural and Political Observations*, p. 21.

52. Ibid., p. 24.

I would like to thank the Carnegie Trust for Scotland for a grant in aid of the research for this chapter.

Index

Age-specific marital fertility
    rates 146
Alcohols 53
Alexandre, Dom Nicholas 93
Almanacs, French 88–9
American settlements, English
    244, 249, 254–5
    deaths from smallpox 250
Anatomy, public interest in
    71–2
Ancien Régime 43
Andriès, Lise 88
Anglo-American social history
    of medicine 38
Annales 4, 15–35
    bio-medical aspects of history
      21
    Braudel as editor 21–3
    decade of 60s 22
    decade of 70s 27–32
    editorial policy 17
    editors 16
    'history of the present' 34
    influence 17
    leitmotifs 16
    longue durée concept 23, 32,
      33, 231, 244, 245
      end of 246
    medical historical articles 19,
      20 (fig), 29–35
    neglect of recent medical
      history 32–3
    nineteenth century history 32
    perspectives 34–5
    preoccupation with pre-
      industrial societies 33–4
    psychiatric articles (1970–75)
      30–1
    special number (1977) 19,
      28–9
Anthropology, history and 90–5
Archaeology of disease 25
Aron, Jean-Paul 21, 27
Asylums 211

casebooks 211
    design in France 31
    York 166–7, 168
Aubrey, John, quoted 249
Aurigemma 31
Avignon medical faculty 59

Baehrel, René 23
Barthez, Pierre-Joseph 68, 70
Bavarian villages 148–9
Becon, Thomas, quoted 236
Belhomme, Jacques 73
Berlin
    mortality 1721–1980 102,
      103 (fig)
    see also Dorotheenstadt parish
Bernard, Jean 31
Bewitchment 92
Bills of mortality 249
Biraben 22
Birth, anthropology of 83
Birth rate, crude (Europe) 133–6
'Black peaks' in population
    development 128
Bleandonu, Gérard 31
Bloch, Marc 16, 19, 82
Body
    disposal of wastes 88
    infants'
      dirtiness 87–8
      fontanelle 87
      washing 87–8
    popular culture and 84–6
Bone-setter 44
Books of health care, French
    88–9
Books of medical recipes,
    French 88–9
Bordeu, Théophile de 70
Bose, Ashish, quoted 126
Bourquenod, Pierre 70–1
Braudel, Fernand 21–2, 23
    death 34
Breastfeeding 139, 150

length in England 139
Bridgewater, Elizabeth,
    Countess of 253
Brittany at end of 18th century
    41–56
    cultural strata 54
    epidemics 49–50
    intendants 45
    medical network 47
    methodological difficulties
        48–51
        demographic 48–50
        retrospective diagnosis of
            disease 50–1
    mortality 41
    parish priest 46
    peasants willing to be bled in
        spring only 52
    popular knowledge of body
        52–5
    population 48
    sources
        advantages/limits 46–8
        proto-statistical era 45
    subsistence crises 49
    unemployment 50
Burke, Peter 30
Burns, relief of pain by blowing
    and praying 93
Burton, Robert 218

Carpentier, Elizabeth 21
Certeau, Michel de 30
Chap-books, French 84, 88–9
Charlatans, 18th–19th century
    74
Charuty, Giordana 91
Chevalier, Louis 33, 38–9
Chicoyneau, Jean François 68
'Chinese' situation (Malthus)
    140, 142
Coherence, divergent logic and
    93–4
Computers, use of, in historical
    research 7, 11, 207, 224–5,
    227, 228–9
Condorcet, Marie Jean,
    Marquis de 72
Consumption, fear of 243

Content, function and 91–2
Corbin, Alain 34
Coroners, courts and records
    215–22
Cullen, William 197 (table),
    200

Death rate, crude (Europe)
    133–6; *see also* Mortality
Dechristianisation of French
    attitudes in 18th century 72
Demographic history 246–8
Demography and qualitative
    history 248–52
Disease, product of faulty
    bodily functioning 72
Diseased limbs not washed 54
Disease-dying-death as
    metaphysical cosmic mental
    pattern 122–5
Divergent logic, coherence and
    93–4
Dorotheenstadt parish (Berlin)
    deaths in 1715–1875 115–22
    causes 116–22
        fever 116–18, 122
        liver diseases 118 (fig),
            121
        old age 120 (fig), 121–2
        teething 119 (fig), 121–2
Dropsy, fear of 243
Dulieu, Louis 59
Duncan, Andrew 195, 197
    (table), 197, 203

Eastern Europe, crude
    birth/death rates 136
Ecole Pratique des Hautes
    Etudes VIe section 21, 27
Edinburgh Royal Infirmary
    176–203
    diagnoses of diseases 178,
        180–1 (table)
        sex differential 182 (table)
        yearly distribution 184
            (table)
    discharges 184–5, 186 (table)
    expenditures for drugs 177
    finances 176–7

hospitalisation 183–4, 185 (table)
management problems 177
mortality rate 185
registers of patients 177–8
servants' ward 182
statistics 177
student casebooks 186–200
  acute/sub-acute/chronic illness 189
  average age of patients 188, 191, 192 (table)
  diagnostic categories and sex distribution 191, 192 (table)
  discharge status 198–9
  duration of complaint before admission 188
  frequency of symptoms 189–90
  medical treatment 191–5
  before admission 189
  occupation of patients 188
  physical methods of treatment 195 (table), 195–7
  presenting symptoms 190–1
  results of medical treatment 197–8, 199 (table)
teaching ward 182
  v. general wards 191
trauma cases 183
venereal disease 179, 183, 184
ward journals 186
Edmundson, Henry, quoted 240–1
Ehrard 23
Empiricism, symbolism and 92–3
England
  crude birth/death rates 135
  expectation of life at birth 136
  in 20th century 143–4
  marshy areas 136, 147, 249
  population growth 136, 142–3, 156
  urban life 142–3
English settlements in America *see* American settlements
Eternity, lost 130
Ethnology 82
European marriage system 144–5
Evelyn, John, death of son 237–8
Expectant mothers' refusals to weigh themselves 85
Expectation of life at birth 133, 136

Fabre, Daniel 91
Family reconstitution 127
Farge, Arlette 24, 29
Faure, Olivier 34
Favret, Jeanne 91, 92
Febvre, Lucien 15–16, 18, 19, 36
Fertility, mortality and living standards 139–42
Fontanelle, cranial 87
Foucault, Michel 2, 24, 37, 75
  history of madness 208
  on medical faculties 58
France
  crude birth/death rates 136
  rural society in 19th century 84–5
Function, content and 91–2

Gainsborough (England), infant mortality 138
Gangrene, fear of 243
Gelfand, Toby, on medical faculties 58
Gélis, Jacques 28, 29, 82
German Empire, infant mortality in 102, 104 (fig)
Gilibert, J.E. 61
Ginzburg, Carlo 83, 91, 232
Gonorrhoea, in 18th century 74
Goubert, Jean-Pierre 22, 27, 28, 29, 34, 36, 40–56
  on historical demography 127

on medical faculties 58
Graunt, John 248, 251–2
Grause, F. 21
Greatrakes, Valentine 245–6
Gregory, James 194–5, 197
(table), 197, 200
Grmek, Mirko 21, 22, 31

Haguenot, Henri 67
Halle, stillbirth, infant/small
children mortality 110
Halliwell, Henry 221
Haparanda 105, 106 (fig)
growth of 107
infant/small child mortality ·
107, 108 (fig)
Hartland (Devon) 137, 144, 147
infant mortality 138
mortality rate 137
Haussmann, Baron, Georges
Eugène 31
Head, dirtiness in infants 88
Health, concern for it in 18th
century 72–3
Historians' prejudices 42–5
Historical methodology in
history of health 40–56
Home, Francis 197 (table), 198
Homeric times, death in 123
(fig)
Honywood, Lady 242
Hope, John 197 (table), 198
Hope, Thomas C. 197, 198,
200
Hôpital Saint-Louis,
Montpellier 70
Hospitals
histories of 175–6; *see also*
Edinburgh Royal
Infirmary
pre-Listerian 3
Hôtel-Dieu Saint-Eloi,
Montpellier 69
public interest in surgery
71–2
Hysteria, female 3

Illich, Ivan 2
Imbert, Jean-François 60, 70

Imhof, Arthur E., afterword
125–31
India, population
studies/sciences 126
Infant mortality 107, 108 (fig),
109 (fig), 110
endogenous/exogenous
causes 109 (fig)
Europe 134
Gainsborough (England) 138
German Empire 102, 104
(fig)
Hartford (Devon) 138
Scandinavia 139
Infusions 53

Josselin, Ralph 241–3, 250

King's Almoner 222

Lactation amenorrhoea
(Sweden) 105, 106 (fig)
Laënnec, Guillaume-Françoise
59, 60, 62, 66, 74
Laget, Mireille 28, 93
La Mettrie 73
Lanteri-Laura, Georges 31
Lebrun, François 58
Le Gaufey, Guy 31
Le Goff, Jacques 21, 22
Leiris, Michel 94, 96–7
Léonard, Jacques 28, 32, 34,
36
Le Père Lachaise cemetery,
Paris 95
Le Roy Ladurie 21, 22, 35–6
Lévi-Strauss, Claude 82, 90
Life-span, average
maximal/actual 129
Longue durée, la 23, 32, 33, 231,
244, 245
end of 246
Lorillot, Dominque 58
Lorraine, O'Donnell 36
Luther, Martin, death of 238

Madhouses, private 73
Madness 207
description of mad people 212

documentary evidence 211
history of 208–10
stereotypes of mental
disorder 213
see also Suicide
Malaria
decline in France 20
effect on marriage 139
Malthus, Thomas R.
(1766–1834) 140, 149, 150
Mandrou, Robert 47
Marriage pattern, European
134
Marshy ground 136, 147, 249
Masonic lodges, French, 18th
century 66
Mass, protest against going to,
during epidemic 54
Maynwaring, Everard 250
Mazaheri 23
Medical advertising in 18th
century 73
Medical anthropology 5
Medical faculties, French 58, 59
Montpellier *see under*
Montpellier medical
students
Medicalisation 2, 57–8, 75
Medical journalism in 18th
century 73
Medical popular books also
cookery books 245
Medical self-publicity in 18th
century 73
Medical therapy, effect on
mortality 143
Melancholy 218
Mentalité 23, 36–7, 238
Mesmerist cult 73
Meyer, Jean 21
Migration 146
Monasteries, French, lunatics
admitted 73
Mondeville, Henri de 83
Montpellier, tourists in 77
Montpellier medical students in
18th century 58–71
antagonism towards surgeons
62–3

botanical gardens restoration
70
clothes 62
courses taken 61
graduates 59, 70–1, 76
Hôpital Saint-Louis,
teaching at 70
Hôtel-Dieu Saint-Eloi,
teaching at 69
licentious behaviour 61–2
medical library 70
pharmaceutical teaching 70
poor quality of teaching
67–8
practical medicine teaching
69–70
private lessons by professors
68–9
professional appointments
63–4
protection of rights 63
public's poor opinion of 60
rivalry with soldiers 62
student councillors 63, 64–5
suspension/restoration/ab-
olition 66
student freemasonry 66
student homesickness 65
student syndics 66
subrogation by professors 68
swordsmanship 62
winter course in anatomy
64
Montpellier physicians 59
Montpellier University 63, 76
archives 77
doctorate in surgery 71, 72
see also Montpellier medical
students
Morelli, Guaberto, death of 237
Mortalities, 'specific' 110–11,
112 (fig), 113 (fig), 114 (fig)
Mortality
England 1550–1800 136–7
underestimation 137–8
urban rates 137
Hartland, Devon 137, 138
infant *see* Infant mortality
west Europe 138–9

Moryson, Fynes 238

Nancy medical faculty 59
Napier, Richard 211–15
Nedertoneå 105, 106 (fig)
    infant/small child mortality
    107, 108 (fig)
Needham, Frederick 166
New Testament-metaphysical
    epoch, death in 123, 128–9
Non-licensed practitioners 74
Non-variables 90–1
North life tables, Princeton
    model 146, 148
Norway, crude birth/death rates
    135

Old Testament times, death in
    123 (fig), 124
Orange medical faculty 59
Overfeeding of hospital patients
    52–3

Paris
    infant mortality in
        neighbouring parishes 148
    medical faculty 58, 59
Parish registrations 249
Pepys, Samuel
    earache 240
    wife's illness 233–5
Perceptions of health and illness
    in early modern England
    231–55
Perkins, William 238, 239
Peter, Jean-Pierre 21–2, 25–7,
    37–8, 83, 95–6
Petonnet, Colette 95
Philadelphia Hospital for the
    Insane 211
Philippsburg
    infant mortality 109 (fig)
    maternal mortality 111, 114
        (fig)
    social inequality and death
        112 (fig)
Philosophe-physician 73
Physician, changing image in
    18th century 76

Plague, explanations of 244
Poor people, threat of
    death/disease in 18th century
    72
Popular knowledge of body
    52–5
Popular medical knowledge
    88–90
Post-metaphysical period, death
    in 123 (fig)
Pouchelle, Marie-Christine 83
Private archives 47
Proverbs, French 84–5, 94

Quacks 44

Recipes in popular medicine,
    French 84, 94
Religious attitudes to illness and
    death 236–9, 248
Remedies of vegetable origin 53
Retreat, The (York) 153–74
    analysis of patients at census
        dates 156
    causes of mental disorder
        165–7
    class distribution of patients
        158
    computation of data 154
    discharges 159
    first admissions 156
    long stay patients 162
    mechanical restraint 163–4
    medical subjects analysed
        155
    medical superintendents 155
    number of patients 156
    outcome of treatment of first
        admissions 169 (table)
    Quaker/non-Quaker patients
        156–8
    qualitative/quantitative
        methods 170–2
    recovery definitions 168–70
    regional institution 157
    seclusion 163–4
    social aspects investigated
        154–5
    subsidised patients 159

women patients 160–2
Revel, Jacques 28, 29
Richard, P. 89
Rigour 94–5
Rituals 92
    trigger of violence in 92
Roche, David 58
Ruffier, Jacques 31
Rumania, birth/death rates 136
Russia, crude birth rate 135

Saint Guéry 53
Saint Méen 53
Saint Rochus 128
Saint Sebastian 128
Saintyves 82
Sauvages, Boissier de 65
Scandinavia, infant mortality
    rate 139
Schmitt, Jean-Claude 82
Schorske, Carl 31
Silences of history 44
'Simples', syrups based on 53
Slack, Paul 251
Sleeping several to a bed 43, 44
Smallpox
    innoculation 74
    more fatal to Indians than
        settlers 250
Société Royale de Médecine 21
Sperber, Dan 91
Spices 53
Star Chamber 222
Strozzi, Allessandra, death of
    son 239
Suicide 207–29
    coroners' records 217–22
        felo de se verdict 218–22
            passim
        non compos mentis verdict
            218–22 *passim*
        returns to King's Bench
            220
    crime in 16th–17th century
        England 218

forfeiture of goods 218,
    221–2
Surgeon(s)
    eighteenth century attitudes
        to 74
    rural practitioners complaints
        80
Surgeon-cum-male-midwife 74
Surgery, public interest in 71–2
Sweden, crude birth/death rates
    135
Symbolism, empiricism and
    92–3
Syphilis, in 18th century 74

Theriac 52

Urban mortality 101–32,
    136–7, 147

Valensi 22
Variation 90–1
Venereal disease, in 18th
    century 73–4
Vermifuges 53
Vess, Donald 58
Vincent 22

Wallington, Nehemiah 239–40
Washing child 87–8
Washing clothes 88
Watching over the dead 53–4
Wesseling, Henk L. 33
'West African' situation 140,
    142
Wet-nurses 87
Willermoz, Pierre-Joseph 70
Winthrop, John 250
Wiseman, John 233–4, 235–6
Witchcraft 92
Wittie, Robert 250, 251
Women midwives 44–5

York Asylum 166–7, 168